Smart Nursing

June Fabre, MBA, RNC, is a premier speaker and educator on nursing management. June Fabre has influenced countless improvements in medical environments that directly affect the careers and lives of nurses, as well as the resulting enhanced patient care. Her books, articles, and workshops synthesize her firsthand experience with nursing challenges in such environments as medical surgical, home care, psychiatry, long-term care, ambulatory care, rehabilitation, and cardiology. Because she has worked as a nurse, educator, and manager, she is uniquely able to see many sides of an issue, whether it's organizational, personal, or academic.

June's mission is to effect positive health care change for its most vital resource—its nurses. She believes that current fears about staffing, financial stress, and patient care can be addressed through the avenue of Smart Nursing. By implementing the Smart Nursing system, organizations across the country are empowering their nurses with the communication and leadership skills that promote a healthy, productive environment.

June Fabre received her RNC and BS in Education from State University College, Plattsburgh, NY; a BSN from Excelsior College, Albany, NY; and her MBA from Plymouth State University, Plymouth, NH. She is a member of the American Organization of Nurse Executives, American Nurses Association, New Hampshire Nurses Association, National Speakers' Association, and Toastmasters International. She has published more than 100 articles in health care journals. For more information, visit www.junefabre.com.

Smart Nursing:

Nurse Retention & Patient Safety Improvement Strategies

SECOND EDITION

JUNE FABRE, MBA, RNC

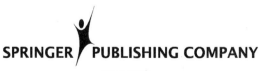

SPRINGER PUBLISHING COMPANY

New York

Springer Publishing Company, LLC
11 West 42nd Street
New York, NY 10036
www.springerpub.com

Acquisitions Editor: Margaret Zuccarini
Production Manager: Kelly J. Applegate
Cover Design: Steve Pisano
Composition: Publication Services
Art: Andrew White

09 10 11 12 13 / 5 4 3 2 1

eBook ISBN: 978-08261-0465-6

Library of Congress Cataloging-in-Publication Data

Fabre, June.
   Smart nursing : nurse retention & patient safety improvement strategies/by June Fabre. — 2nd ed.
      p. ; cm.
   Includes bibliographical references and index.
   ISBN 978-0-8261-0464-9 (pbk.)
   1. Nursing services—United States—Personnel management.   2. Nursing services—United States—Administration.   3. Nurses—Supply and demand—United States.   4. Nurses—Recruiting—United States.   5. Nursing errors—United States—Prevention.   I. Title.
   [DNLM: 1. Nursing—organization & administration.   2. Job Satisfaction. 3. Medical Errors—prevention & control.   4. Nurse-Patient Relations.   5. Patient Satisfaction. WY 105 F123s 2008]
   RT89.3.F33 2008
   610.73068'3—dc22   2008040793

Printed in the United States of America by Bang Printing.

To My Parents
Fritz Bendel and Olga Bendel, LPN (retired),
who lived and loved the American Dream.

Contents

Contributors

Beth Boynton, RN, MS
Nurse Trainer, Coach, Consultant, Speaker
www.bethboynton.com
York Beach, Maine

Jeanette Ives Erickson, RN, MS
Senior Vice President, Patient Care; Chief Nurse
Massachusetts General Hospital
Boston, Massachusetts

Kristin L. Gillen, MSN, RN
Director of Nursing
Renown Health
Reno, Nevada

Diana Halfer, MSN, RN, NE-BC
Administrator, Clinical and Organizational Development
Children's Memorial Medical Center
Chicago, Illinois

Susan Hoolahan, RN, MSN, CNAA-BC
Vice President of Patient Care Services, CNO
University of Pittsburgh Medical Center, UPMC-St Margaret
Pittsburgh, Pennsylvania

Jacqueline O'Brien, MSN, RN, CIC
Director of Nursing Education
University of Pittsburgh Medical Center, UPMC-St Margaret
Pittsburgh, Pennsylvania

Linda Pullins, RN, BS
Vice President, Patient Care Services
Marion General Hospital
Marion, Ohio

Patricia Byrnes Schmehl, RN, MSN
Administrator, Women's Services
Inova Fairfax Hospital Women's Center
Falls Church, Virginia

Foreword

Smart Nursing: Nurse Retention and Patient Safety Improvement Strategies, Second Edition, features an expanded Smart Nursing model, with a new chapter on caring; additions to evidence-based practice, integrating new Magnet and Joint Commission initiatives; and updated recent health care and business best practices. Smart Nursing continues to assist clinical nurses and managers with realistic strategies to prevent chronic understaffing, improve patient safety, and build a case for retaining a stable nursing staff, including success stories from nurses and managers around the country.

Smart Nursing, Second Edition gives even more reasons for viewing nurses as invaluable assets in multiple health care settings and expands the leadership chapter to include leadership roles for nurses who are not managers. Ideas for improving collaboration with other nurses, physicians, managers, and other departments add to its overall approach to changing the health care system to one in which individual caring nurses can practice in a supportive, appreciative environment.

New worksheets, exercises, and models have been added, along with expanded strategies for education and communication so that students, new graduates, and veteran nurses can function in the workplace with greater respect, autonomy, and satisfaction. *Smart Nursing* continues to recommend the reclaiming of core values, such as integrity, flexibility, and caring, and combines them with other initiatives, such as creating a just culture and practicing lean strategies.

We need the participation of nurses at every level to change a system that has not performed for patients, staff, or management. *Smart*

Nursing, Second Edition provides the tools for nurses and managers to communicate effectively, work together, and collaborate on a new vision for health care.

Margaret A. Fitzgerald, DNP, FNP-BC, FAANP, CSP
President, Fitzgerald Health Education Associates, Inc.
North Andover, MA
Family Nurse Practitioner, Adjunct Faculty,
Family Practice Residency Program
Greater Lawrence (MA) Family Health Center

Acknowledgments

Writing a book is a process that requires the assistance of others, and I would like to recognize the people who have helped me along the way.

A special thank-you to all of the members of the Derry Writers Group, especially Janet Buell, J. Richard Reed, Roger Davies, Dennis Hett, Marilyn Pontuck, Marilyn McNamara, and Joe Smiga. J. Richard Reed invited me to the Derry Writers Group, where I learned to write for publication. I'd also like to express my appreciation to the Author's Guild and the New Hampshire Writers Project for the support and education that they provide to authors.

I'd like to thank my colleagues at the National Speakers Association, especially Dianna Booher, MA, CSP, CPAE, Booher Consultants Inc.; Dr. Margaret A. Fitzgerald, DNP, FNP-BC, NP-C, FAANP, CSP President, Fitzgerald Health Education Associates, Inc.; W. Mitchell, CPS, CSP, CPAE; Steve Lishansky, CEO of OPTIMIZE International; Captain Larry Brudnicki, Perfect Storm Solutions; and Susan Keane Baker, MHA, Speaking of Exceptional Patient Care. And I would also like to thank every single member of the National Speakers Association–New England for their continuous caring, warm support, and loyal friendship for more than 10 years.

I appreciate those who generously contributed to *Smart Nursing*: Beth Boynton, RN, MS; Jeanette Ives Erickson, RN, MS; Kristin L. Gillen, MSN, RN; Diana Halfer, MSN, RN, NE-BC; Susan Hoolahan, RN, MSN, CNAA-BC; Jacqueline O'Brien, MSN, RN, CIC; Linda Pullins, RN, BS; and Patricia Byrnes Schmehl, RN, MSN.

Various nurses read portions of my manuscript, suggested examples to use, or assisted me in determining the best way to present important nursing issues. These wonderful nurses are Jean Watson, Joanne Tethers, Claudia Cunningham, Suzanne Belanger, Anne Smith, Gerri Gowlis, Marilyn Asselin, Byrdie Jo Baker, Laura Rapp, Deborah O'Neil, Louise McGourty, Sigrid Kuriger, Yvette Moquin, Elaine St. Pierre,

Jill Ellis, Marie Loignon, Joyce Raguse, and my sister, Joan Livingston. Their education and experience include LPN, RN, RN BC, ARNP, MSN, MBA, and PhD. Their broad perspectives have helped me reach my goal—that *Smart Nursing* should provide information and support to all nurses.

I also thank librarians Ruslyn Vear, Head of Reference Services, and Sarah Leonardi, Reference Librarian, at the Amherst Town Library, and Dorothy Y. Kameoka, from the Dorothy M. Breene Memorial Library, who helped a great deal with my research. And I appreciate the editorial suggestions that I received from Prill McGann, Janice Borzandowski, Jean Rogers, and my editor at Springer, Margaret Zuccarini.

My three daughters and their families were patient and encouraging, and have helped me maintain my sense of humor: Michelle, Jim, and Lucas Roberge, Kim Fabre and Chris Williams, and Sherri Fabre and Andy White. I also appreciate the warm support and guidance of Rev. Susan A. Henderson and the members of the Women's Spirituality Group at the Amherst Congregational Church.

To the members of the American Organization of Nurse Executives, the Massachusetts Organization of Nurse Executives, the American Nurses Association, the New Hampshire Nurses Association, and the members of Manchester Toastmasters, I appreciate your friendship and leadership role modeling.

Why Use Smart Nursing?

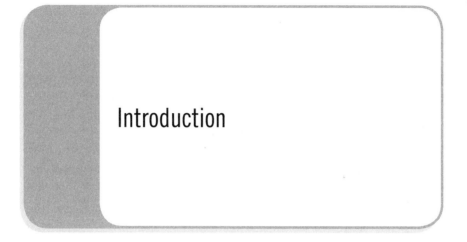

Introduction

In the children's story, "Jack and the Beanstalk," the mythical beanstalk grows and allows Jack to enter a mysterious world of peril and adventure, the land of the giant and his extraordinary riches. Within this land is a goose that lays golden eggs.

Health care managers face a similar situation. They also live with peril and adventure, especially while staffing their facilities. They have golden geese but don't always recognize them. Their golden geese come disguised as nurses. Organizations are figuratively killing their nurses, with negative working conditions and by actively ignoring their contributions. Nurses are one of health care's greatest assets—health care gold.

In the 1990s, health care management slashed staff instead of performing the precise surgery needed to decrease waste. Nurses could not survive in this new environment of overuse, so they either burned out or found other careers. Now, health care facilities face sinking financial futures because of the nursing shortage. Nursing costs have increased, and some facilities have been forced to put expansion plans on hold. Bottom lines have declined, and facilities have not been able to offer necessary services to their communities.

I believe that caring people, not policies and procedures, determine whether patients receive quality health care services. Many of these caring people are nurses. Unfortunately, the nursing shortage threatens worldwide health care systems. An article in *The Wall Street Journal* cited a study from the *New England Journal of Medicine* (Needleman, Beurhaus, Mattke, Stewart, & Zelevinsky, 2002) in highlighting the seriousness of this shortage: "When there are too few registered nurses at bedsides, patients are significantly more likely to suffer serious complications, such as urinary-tract infections, internal bleeding, and even death" (as cited in Johannes, 2002). Moreover, nurses are being overworked yet underutilized, ignored, and even censured for speaking up; the result is that patient safety is being compromised. An editorial in *The New York Times*, referring to a report in the *Journal of the American Medical Association* (Aiken, Clarke, Silbur, & Sloane, 2003), addressed this aspect of the problem:

> When hospital nurses are given too many patients to care for, the patients have a much greater risk of dying. Adding a single patient to a nurse's caseload seems to increase the risk of dying within 30 days by 7 percent.

The National Patient Safety Foundation attributes the medical error crisis to an inability to overcome systems problems, exacerbated by the growing complexity in health care, which requires improved communication and cooperation among health care professionals (www.npsf.org).

Nurses need greater power, respect, and communication expertise to overcome these systems problems. A lack of courtesy and respect can chip away at a nurse's sense of self, destroying his or her energy level and motivation. Nurses become dispirited when system delays cause medical errors and deaths despite the best efforts of the nursing staff.

Anita L. Tucker describes the performance degradation of nurses caused by operational failures. In this research, Tucker defines operational failures as errors in the supply of necessary material or information and as obstacles that "can frustrate and hinder employees, decreasing individual and organizational performance" (Tucker, 2004). These operational failures intensify health care costs and staffing shortages. Tucker provides us with the following challenge: [operational failures] "illuminate opportunities for improvement."

We can turn our health care problems into opportunities, and this is one of the purposes of Smart Nursing. Smart Nursing harmonizes well with standards from the Joint Commission, the forces of magnetism from the American Nurse Credentialing Center (ANCC), and with "lean" management strategies. This book, *Smart Nursing*, describes practical techniques that every nurse, manager, and organization can use to restore patient safety, reduce nurse turnover, and stimulate realistic health care solutions. Throughout, solid data from business and health care sources are used, yet the book is written in an easy-to-understand style, to ensure its accessibility to readers: chief nurses, managers, registered nurses (RNs), licensed practical nurses (LPNs); non-nurse professionals such as physicians, chief executive officers (CEOs), or trustees; or consumers who are interested in learning how to improve health care. Smart Nursing assists nurses and managers in how to work together, using conceptual, communication, and leadership approaches. The wisdom behind these strategies is that they blend health care knowledge with business expertise.

THE SEVEN CORE VALUES OF SMART NURSING

The seven core values of Smart Nursing—caring, respect, simplicity, flexibility, integrity, professional culture, and communication—cost nothing. However, they are essential for patient safety and quality. More than helping nurses to maximize the "nursing process" with commitment,

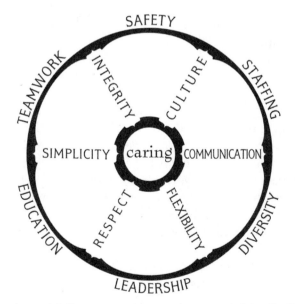

The *Smart Nursing* model. Seven core values—caring, respect, integrity, flexibility, simplicity, professional culture, and communication—form the structure and strength of Smart Nursing.

competence, and compassion, Smart Nursing addresses the bottom line for managers. In short, the dollar difference between the present level of nurse productivity and a nurse's full professional capacity is the potential cost savings that Smart Nursing offers.

Smart Nursing identifies 10 guiding principles of Smart Health Care Management, promoting the wholeness of the health care system. These principles assist organizations to synergize components of good management practice.

THE 10 GUIDING PRINCIPLE OF SMART HEALTH CARE MANAGEMENT

1. Nurses are an essential part of a health care facility's investment.
2. Systems problems prevent nurses from performing at their full professional capacity.
3. Restoring the value of nursing by considering nurses as assets and treating them as valued professionals maximizes the return on an organization's human resource investment.
4. Organizations that provide environments where nurses can perform at their best attract and retain the best people.
5. Leaders and managers are more effective when they build strong relationships with their staff.
6. Long-term strategies such as effective communication and staff-friendly cultures enable organizations to achieve the best results.
7. Combining sound clinical practices with ethical business actions produces the safest and most cost-effective patient care.
8. Positive relationships among health care professionals generate energy and raise productivity.
9. Clinical nurses who can make decisions at the patient level save management time and increase patient satisfaction.
10. Individuals who embrace lifelong learning develop the ability to thrive in a rapidly changing world.

Organizations often justify their treatment of nurses by suggesting that financial constraints are forcing their actions, but research and experiential data show the opposite. The Advisory Board in Washington, D.C., estimates that a 500-bed hospital can save $800,000 a year by cutting its nurse turnover by a mere 3% (Nursing Executive Center, 2000).

CONCEPTUAL FRAMEWORK OF SMART NURSING

Smart Nursing and the nursing process are based on general systems theory, which researchers discovered years ago to be the most effective way to study human processes in fields such as psychology, sociology, and political science. General systems theory seeks to understand the "wholeness" of any system by understanding the interdependence of its parts.

Too many health care organizations are using short-term fixes—Band-Aid solutions—that exacerbate the nursing shortage. It is the long-term strategies of Smart Nursing, such as building relationships and effective communication, that deliver better results.

I propose a new mind-set: one that views nurses not by the number of tasks that they can complete, but as important professionals with invaluable insights and an immeasurable capacity to care.

Everyone—the consumer, the business executives, the government, and the nursing community itself—is alarmed at the high rate of medical errors and our failing health care system. Now is the right time for change. Now is the right time for nurses and managers to learn to work together. And now is the right time for health care organizations to take better care of one of their most important asserts—their nurses.

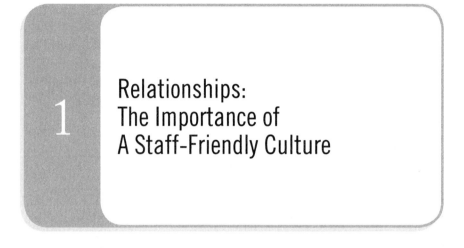

Relationships:
The Importance of
A Staff-Friendly Culture

The key to unleashing the organization's potential to excel is putting that power in the hands of the people who perform the work. **—*James M. Kouzes***

You, the nurse manager, arrive at your office at 8:00 on Monday morning. Stephanie, one of your most competent nurses, asks for a few minutes of your time. She hands you a letter of resignation. She is the third RN to do so in the last 60 days.

Even as you consider ways to fill the holes in the schedule, you wonder why she is leaving. After all, the nurses have just received a substantial pay raise, and they have the best benefits package in the area. Managers and non-nurses remark that the nurses are getting everything they want but never seem to be satisfied.

As for yourself, you must address what is becoming a vicious cycle of nurse resignations and overtime for the remaining staff, which you know will lead to more nurse burnout and more resignations.

But from Stephanie's point of view, the reasons she resigned are all too apparent. Consider how one of her workdays develops:

1. She arrives for work and discovers that she will be short-staffed.
2. During the course of the day, she encounters disrespectful behavior and asks herself why she bothers. The sources of this disrespectful behavior are usually physicians, managers, or other

nurses. Patients are usually the prime source of support that nurses receive.

3.   She has no time for a break because of the heavy workload, causing her to be exhausted early and less effective as the day wears on.

4.   During a staff meeting, she makes some suggestions that would improve care, but management tables them, leaving her frustrated and angry.

5.   There are several patient admissions that afternoon, but the staff has the attitude of "every nurse for herself," each struggling to finish her work and unwilling to lend a hand where it's needed.

At the end of the day, certain tasks that would have made a big difference to patients remain undone, and Stephanie leaves work feeling that the patients received poor care. In sum, it was another in a long series of *energy-draining* days that add up to Stephanie's decision to finally throw in the towel.

It doesn't have to be like this. In a staff-friendly culture, nurses have a completely different experience—an *energy-enhancing* experience. Though their workload is substantial, they find they can do it effectively and efficiently. They are treated as important professionals. They can say, and mean, "We don't do rude here." Their suggestions at the last staff meeting have been given full consideration and will be implemented the same week. They feel they are part of a high-performance team, one that can handle multiple admissions easily by working cooperatively. They feel good physically as well, because despite the heavy activity on the unit, they are encouraged to make time for meals and breaks. Thus, they leave work tired but satisfied, safe in the knowledge that their hard work had meaning and resulted in excellent patient care.

Nurses are your organization's best revenue sources. Nurses *generate revenue* by delivering excellent patient care. When patients choose a health care facility, they want safety and a personal connection with staff members; nurses satisfy both of these needs.

Nurses generate revenue when their personal connections keep patients coming back to your facility. These connections do not necessarily take a lot of time. It is not the time that's important; it is the quality of the connections and the skill with which they are made.

For example: While preparing to perform an admission assessment, a nurse notices that the patient is having an important conversation with a family member. She shows compassion by telling the patient she will return in 15 minutes for the assessment. Time spent: 30 seconds. The result is invaluable patient appreciation and satisfaction. This provides a source for future revenue flow.

Staffing issues are more easily resolved in a staff-friendly culture because there is a spirit of collaboration, humor, and cooperation.

For example: A nurse wants to avoid working a weekend double shift. As she and several peers wait for the weekly staff meeting to begin, she asks one of them to substitute for her, commenting, "I will be so sad if you can't do it." She uses the opportunity for some humorous persuasion as well. She turns to another peer and says, "Do you want to see how sad we will be if you don't work on Saturday? See our sad faces!" The staff has a good belly laugh, and the nurse successfully covers the shift. And the shift is covered at straight time, not premium pay, so it turns out to be a money-saving solution as well.

Staff-friendly cultures are very cost effective because staff can spend 100% of their time and energy doing their work instead of wasting time and energy surviving a dysfunctional system. If a nurse earns $50,000 but has to waste 25% of her time dealing with unnecessary conflict and petty political agendas, you lose $12,500 of the nursing value for each nurse. With only 16 nurses, that adds up to a lost value of $200,000 a year. And the negative culture decreases nurse satisfaction and increases staff turnover. The cost of staff turnover can add hundreds of thousands of dollars to that $200,000. Can we afford to continue wasting nurse resources this way?

A Long-Term Perspective

Long-term strategies prevail in staff-friendly cultures. Long-term strategies of respect, relationships, and collaboration provide an environment where staff can thrive. These long-term strategies can transform our current health care environment from chaos into an environment of consistent quality and safety.

According to a 2006 honesty and ethics Gallup poll, people respect nurses more highly than any other profession; 84% gave nurses the highest score (Gallup, 2008). Health care organizations should show respect for nurses by giving them the power to control their practice, the credit for their accomplishments, and the opportunity to utilize their full professional capacity.

One solution to the nursing shortage is to educate more nurses. But research about new nurses indicates that ethical issues and general working conditions can be linked to job dissatisfaction and can lead to the high turnover rate of nurses (55%–61%) within their first year of practice and suggests that it is beneficial for health care institutions to retain these nurses because high turnover is expensive (West, 2007). Another article, this one from *Nursing Economics*, also indicates a new nurse turnover rate as high as 61% (Pine & Tart, 2007).

Managers and nurses build relationships that matter when they consistently practice honesty and trust and offer praise for work well done. Health care is a relationship business. It is built on relationships between caregivers and patients, as well as on relationships between caregivers and health care providers. However, nursing productivity is often measured only in the number of tasks that a nurse can accomplish, which is like going to the store and buying apples and then trying to judge your success by counting how many oranges you have.

Many facilities rely heavily on sign-on bonuses and optimistic recruitment ads. These techniques attract nurses to the facility, but those same nurses usually leave when their commitment expires. Or they resign when they realize that the facility wasn't all it had been described to be. These are short-term fixes.

Consider the folly of too many quick fixes. Suppose a two-year-old has a tantrum. Occasionally giving in to a child's demands probably won't cause any harm. However, using the quick fix and always giving in to those demands produces a monster. Health care has created its own monster by using the quick fix much too often. This Band-Aid approach has left a reservoir of unresolved issues: frustrated and burned-out employees, dissatisfied patients, and wasted resources.

Nurse retention improves when managers put Smart Nursing core values and guiding principles into practice. Patients are safer when nurses who are reporting safety concerns are viewed as credible reporters and when patients know that reporting those concerns results in positive action, not retaliation.

Reducing complications and unnecessary deaths, of course, benefits patients and their families. But it also benefits health care facilities, because it improves their reputation. With more patients, revenue increases, improving the bottom line. Nurses are renewable resources with substantial value, but not when management burns them out.

Ann O'Sullivan, MSN, RN, testifying before the Senate Governmental Affairs Committee on behalf of the American Nurses' Association, had this to say:

> Nurses are, understandably, reluctant to accept positions in which they will face inappropriate staffing, be confronted by mandatory overtime,

inappropriately rushed through patient care activities and face retaliation if they report unsafe practices. (O'Sullivan, 2001)

Nurses are powerless. Even during nursing shortages, facilities waste nurses. They waste nursing time, ignore nursing potential, and destroy nursing spirit. Many organizations value tasks but ignore nurses' ideas and opinions.

For example, a nurse observes symptoms of physical decline in a patient—the patient's respiratory rate is 40, but the normal respiratory rate for an adult is 20. The nurse's assessment rules out hyperventilation and anxiety, which, if present, would indicate less significant reasons for rapid respirations. This nurse is very concerned that the patient is having early symptoms of a major medical problem and reports these observations to the charge nurse, supervisor, and physician. The nurse asks for additional diagnostic tests to be done. The request is denied, and no one takes action. Nurses only have the power to continue assessing and reporting, not to order additional diagnostic tests or medication. Eventually, after repeated requests, the patient goes into cardiac arrest; the rest of the team finally jumps into action. Additional testing is finally done during the resuscitation process, but it is too late, and the patient dies. This is an example of a "failure to rescue" event, as described in recent research (Needleman, Buerhaus, Mattke, Stewart, & Zeleuinsky, 2002). In this case, the nurse had recognized the symptoms early, but those who had the power to act did not take those early symptoms seriously.

In the midst of the nursing shortage, nurses often don't even have the extra time for frequent patient assessments. For example, a patient's medical order may require assessment of vital signs every 4 hours. But if a nurse is concerned about a patient's condition, he or she may want to recheck the patient's vital signs every 30 minutes for a short while. However, with a heavy nursing assignment, there may be no time to follow through on more frequent checks of vital signs. Other responsibilities (treatments and medications) consume all of the nurse's time, so he or she may miss the early symptoms of major complications.

Patients appreciate nurses' compassion because it contributes so much quality to their health care services, but others disregard it. Nursing management has little influence in the power game, and this leaves nurses with no voice at all.

Clinical nurses and managers need to teach others how to treat them with respect. There are various ways to accomplish this, and your choices depend on your own personal style.

■ Be assertive about ending disrespectful behavior. If someone is rude, bring it to his or her attention assertively and make it clear that disrespectful behavior is not tolerated.

■ Insist that supervisors and physicians take timely action when you notice that a patient is in physical decline. It is unacceptable for patients to suffer with unnecessary medical decline.

■ Document everything that you do and say accurately, completely, and professionally.

■ Take appropriate pride in the skillful assessments and astute observations that prevent patients from having unnecessary physical decline. Patients usually acknowledge your value, but managers and physicians frequently do not.

Nurses may need more staff or updated equipment, but they may be preempted by the budgetary requests of those with more power. Because money is scarce, nursing input often is *not* viewed as a priority and is therefore the last request to be taken into consideration.

Management and physicians often hear reports of valid problems and treat them as complaints. Whistle-blowers are treated harshly. In their 2001 study of nurses, Harvard researchers (Tucker, Edmonson, & Spear) observed the difficulty that nurses encountered when they tried to report significant information:

> We did not observe any instances where the nurse contacted someone about a trivial or insignificant exception. In fact, we observed several occasions where we were surprised that the nurse did *not* raise awareness around a problem that we felt could have serious consequences.

When nurses are concerned about a patient's physical decline, they are often disregarded, even if they express their concern through the proper channels. Nurses can't call physicians who work in the emergency room, because it is against protocol. The protocol represents a valid and safe system in most cases. Physicians, as independent practitioners or as part of a group practice, do not usually examine each other's patients unless there is a conversation between them first. Many times, when this conversation happens, an order is written, arranging for examination of the patient, and the patient then receives the necessary care.

When the conversation doesn't happen, nurses can be left with a deteriorating patient and no way to intervene. In such cases, the patient would receive better care anyplace *except* in a hospital. Consider how one patient was denied proper care in the following example.

In one instance, several concerned nurses tried to facilitate a physician-to-physician conversation so that the emergency room physician could examine an inpatient who was in physical decline. During one of these situations, a very frustrated nurse suggested humorously to a colleague, "Why don't we get the patient dressed, put him in a wheelchair, and then wheel him into the emergency room's front door with the following comment: 'We found this guy lying outside in the parking lot. He looks sick. Can you check him over?'" Such humor releases stress when nurses are powerless.

This problem has been partially addressed by using hospitalists, physicians whose job responsibilities include examining hospitalized patients. However, not all hospitals use hospitalists, and not all physicians ask them to care for their patients.

Other situations reveal the way that vital nursing observation builds partnerships with physicians. For instance, a nurse looked at a physician order that seemed different than usual. After she called the physician and read the order, the physician said, "Thank-you for *thinking*. This order is wrong." The physician corrected the order, and a potential medication error was averted. It's that easy. Simple respectful conversations are one of the ways to prevent serious medical errors. Why don't we use this method more often?

Health Care Problems Are Opportunities

Problems are one side of the health care coin, but there are also opportunities—opportunities to improve the care that staff nurses, managers, and physicians provide.

Smart Nursing adds to nurse effectiveness with strategies for critical thinking, assertiveness, leadership, and communication. Public speaking and writing for publication are also an important part of the mix. With Smart Nursing, nurses learn to describe their full professional value quantitatively as well as qualitatively.

Workloads for health care professionals will not decline. If anything, they will increase. But Smart Nursing core values and guiding principles enable nurses to manage heavy workloads without burnout. Smart Nursing enables the whole medical team to work in synergy within a positive work environment. A positive environment is the foundation of high productivity, because it allows staff to access their higher selves. You have probably had experience using your higher self during particularly harmonious periods of your life. Think back to when you were working on a project that you especially enjoyed. Recall your energy level. You wanted to spend more time on your project, didn't you? And the time that you spent working seemed more like play than like work. You were accessing your higher self and therefore capable of achieving more work than usual. It's the same for nurses working in a staff-friendly culture. Contrast this experience to a time when you were involved in unsatisfactory work. Time dragged, and you felt like procrastinating and putting the work off as long as possible. That's how our present atmosphere saps nurse productivity.

Gary Zukav puts it this way in his book, *The Seat of the Soul*: "When we align our thoughts, emotions and actions with the highest part of ourselves, we are filled with enthusiasm, purpose and meaning. Life is rich and full . . . We are joyously and intimately engaged with our world" (Zukav, 1989).

Are you interested in learning how to turn the nursing crisis into an opportunity to improve patient care? With Smart Nursing, you can improve the treatment of nurses and improve medical care for yourself, your loved ones, and your community.

BEST PRACTICE: A NURSE LEADER IN ACTION

Jeanette Ives Erickson, RN, MS, senior vice president for patient care and chief nurse, Massachusetts General Hospital, Boston, MA

Building Bridges: A Strategy for Success

As the chief nurse of the Massachusetts General Hospital, I am surrounded by the best and brightest clinical nurses and leadership in nursing. I believe the reason for our success is that we always remember why we became nurses. Our commitment to nursing has guided us in creating an agenda for MGH nursing that is aligned with our own personal values and passion for the profession.

Three Cornerstones for Success

When I assumed the role of chief nurse, I immediately worked with my leadership team to create the three cornerstones for MGH nursing: a shared vision, guiding principles, and long-term strategic goals.

1. **Shared vision:** We hold a shared picture of the future that we seek to create.

2. **Value statements or guiding principles:** We believe in the worth of what we have and [in] our desire to create something new. Our value statements influence strategic planning because they are the result of staff decisions and behaviors. The true test of our values occurs when our staff—and, more important, our patients—can see and feel those values in action.

3. **Long-term strategic goals:** Long-term objectives are the measure of departmental and organizational effectiveness. They are not quick fixes. They are high-leverage, long-term strategies that create fundamental change and solutions.

Create Bridges Between Management and Nursing

These three cornerstones paved the way for strategic planning. I have seen many strategic plans end up in colorful binders with great graphics, but covered with dust from lack of use. They do not come alive. I was committed to making certain that MGH nursing's strategic plan came alive.

I see strategic planning as an opportunity to create a bridge between clinical nurses and management. Both management and clinical nurses are necessary to fulfill our vision. Clinical nurses have both formal and informal opportunities to provide input into the strategic plan and to assess how it's going.

Examples of How We Create Bridges

1. I meet with a staff nurse representative from every clinical unit each month at our Staff Nurse Advisory Committee. This committee forms a bridge between clinical nurses and management so that we can work together as partners to solve health care dilemmas.

2. We use an annual survey called the Staff Perception Survey of Professional Practice Environment. The survey is sent to clinical nurses throughout MGH and queries them about their feelings of autonomy, control over practice, collaborative relationships, and perceptions about what's working and what's not working.

3. Through ongoing staff forums and clinical rounds, staff members can voice their perceptions about their practice.

4. We obtain leadership input through formal meetings and quarterly retreats in which we critically review where we are going and how we are going to get there.

Prepare Staff for Strategic Planning

Our strategic plan resonates with both clinical nurses and leadership because their voices are heard and incorporated into it. We make an investment of time and energy to prepare staff to be able to participate actively in strategic planning. However, the dividends are high. Every member of the Department of Nursing feels ownership of our strategic direction. And clinical nurses and leadership see evidence that they are being heard because the strategic plan is written in their words. Together, we translate the plan into action.

The following are the vision statement, guiding principles, and long-term strategic goals that we generated at MGH:

Vision Statement

As nurses, health professionals, and patient-care-services support staff, our every action is guided by knowledge, enabled by skill, and motivated by compassion. Patients are our primary focus, and the way in which we deliver care reflects that focus every day. We believe in creating a practice environment that has no barriers, that is built on a spirit of inquiry, and that reflects a culturally competent workforce supportive of the patient-focused values of this institution. It is through our professional practice model that we make our vision a demonstrable truth every day—by letting our thoughts, decisions, and actions be guided by our values. As clinicians, we ensure that our practice is caring, innovative, scientific, and empowering and that it is based on a foundation of leadership and entrepreneurial teamwork.

Guiding Principles

We are ever alert for opportunities to improve patient care; we provide care based on the latest **research findings**.

We recognize the importance of **encouraging** patients and families to participate in the decisions affecting their care.

We are most effective as a team; we continually strengthen our relationships with each other and actively promote **diversity** within our staff.

We enhance patient care and the systems supporting that care as we work with others; we eagerly enter new **partnerships** with people inside and outside the Massachusetts General Hospital.

We never lose sight of the needs and expectations of our patients and their families as we make clinical decisions based on the most **effective** use of internal and external resources.

We view **learning** as a lifelong process that is essential to the growth and development of clinicians who are striving to deliver quality patient care.

We acknowledge that maintaining the **highest standards** of patient-care delivery is a never-ending process that involves patients, family, nurses, all health care providers, and the community at large.

Long-Term Strategic Goals

Enhance communication to promote employees' understanding of organizational imperatives and their involvement in clinical decisions that affect their practice.

Promote and advance a professional practice model that is responsive to the essential requirements of the patients, the staff, and the organization.

Ensure appropriate allocation of resources and equitable, competitive salaries.

Position nurses, therapists, social workers, and chaplains to have a strong voice in issues affecting patient-care outcomes.

Provide quality patient care within a cost-effective delivery system.

Lead initiatives that foster diversity of staff and create culturally competent care strategies that support both the local and the international patients whom we serve.

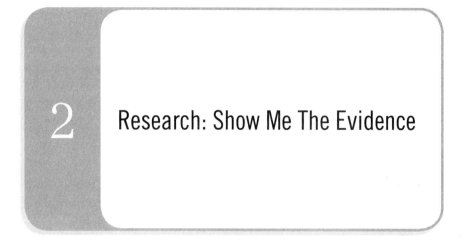

2 Research: Show Me The Evidence

Research is formalized curiosity. It is poking and prying with a purpose.
—*Zora Neale Hurston*

SHOW ME THE EVIDENCE

Health care is shifting its perspective; we now ask, "What is the evidence?" before committing to a course of action.

The following is a review of significant research studies about the nursing shortage. I have included three types of research: clinical, organizational, and financial.

The current nursing shortage is different from prior nursing shortages experienced from time to time. Nurses have been complaining about short staffing for a long time. Studies undertaken at the end of the 1990s confirmed what nurses feared the most: there is a strong correlation between the number of patients cared for by each registered nurse and the number of patient complications and deaths. Even one extra patient added to a nurse's assignment severely interferes with patient safety.

Studies about workplace environments show that nurses are routinely ignored and treated with disrespect. Nurses have frequently described how disrespectful behavior has interfered with their ability to fulfill their patient care responsibilities and to enjoy the same level of professional respect as others.

Managers have stated that nurse staffing cuts have been necessary to balance the budget. Yet studies examining the cost of the nursing crisis have shown that the costs of high nursing turnover exceed the cost of maintaining a stable and adequate nursing staff.

Clinical Research

Excerpts follow from the abstract from one of the largest clinical studies about the nursing crisis:

How the Study Was Done

We used administrative data from 1997 for 799 hospitals in 11 states (covering 5,075,969 discharges of medical patients and 1,104,659 discharges of surgical patients) to examine the relation between the amount of care provided by nurses at the hospital and patients' outcomes. We conducted regression analyses, in which we controlled for patients' risk of adverse outcomes, differences in the nursing care needed for each hospital's patients, and other variables.

Conclusions

A higher proportion of hours of nursing care provided by registered nurses and a greater number of hours of care by registered nurses per day are associated with better care for hospitalized patients [. . .] "Hospitals," wrote Lewis Thomas in *The Youngest Science*, are "held together, glued together, enabled to function [. . .] by the nurses" (Thomas, 1995).

As hospitals have responded to financial pressure from Medicare, managed care, and other private payers, registered nurses have become increasingly dissatisfied with the working conditions in hospitals.

Among medical patients, we found an association between registered-nurse staffing and six outcomes. Both a higher proportion of licensed-nurse care provided by registered nurses [. . .] and more registered-nurse-hours per day [. . .] were associated with a shorter length of stay and lower rates of urinary tract infections and upper gastrointestinal bleeding. A higher proportion of registered-nurse-hours [. . .] but not a greater number of registered-nurse-hours per day [. . .] was associated with lower rates of three other adverse outcomes: pneumonia, shock, or cardiac arrest, and failure to rescue.

Among surgical patients, a higher proportion of registered-nurse-hours [. . .] was associated with a lower rate of urinary tract infection. A greater number of registered-nurse-hours per day [. . .] was associated with a lower rate of failure to rescue.

A greater number of licensed-nurse-hours per day was associated with a shorter length of stay among medical patients.

Our findings clarify the relation between the level of staffing by nurses and the quality of care. We found consistent evidence of an association between higher levels of staffing by registered nurses and lower rates of adverse outcomes. (Needleman, Buerhaus, Mattke, Stewart, & Zelevinsky, 2002)

According to *The Wall Street Journal,* "A new study shows that inadequate nursing care can cause devastating problems for patients [. . .] the findings, which come amid a prolonged nursing shortage, suggest that patients should consider how many registered nurses are on hand when choosing a hospital" (Johannes, 2002).

An Institute of Medicine report concluded six years ago that there were not enough data to show that more nurses improve patients' medical outcomes. Today's study, which is based on six million patient records [. . .] finally provides the proof [that] having a higher proportion of registered nurses in the total nursing-staff mix noticeably improved care. (Johannes, 2002)

A clinical study from Pennsylvania came to the following conclusions:

Aiken and colleagues linked information from nurse surveys, hospital administrative sources, and hospital discharge summaries to examine whether hospital nurse staffing and educational level are associated with differences in the outcomes of surgical patients.

- The investigators used data from 168 non-federal general hospitals in Pennsylvania, surveys of 10,184 nurses, and information from 232,342 general, orthopedic, and vascular surgery patients.
- After adjusting for many hospital and patient factors, nurse staffing was associated with significant increases in 30-day mortality and failure to rescue. The results suggest that every additional patient in a nurse's workload increases the odds of patient mortality by 7%.
- The investigators estimate that the risk of death was 14% higher in hospitals where the nurse's average workload was 6 patients or more, and 31% higher in hospitals with workloads of 8 patients or more, compared to hospitals where nurses cared for 4 or fewer patients.

■ A direct comparison of staffing hospitals uniformly at 8 vs. 4 patients per nurse yielded estimates of 5 excess deaths per 1,000 patients, and 18 excess deaths per 12,000 patients with complications.

■ Having found an association between nurse staffing and patient outcomes, the investigators analyzed whether other nurse characteristics, such as years of experience or educational level, are associated with mortality rates [. . .]

■ Nurses' educational level was strongly associated with mortality. The authors estimate that the odds of 30-day mortality and failure to rescue would be 19% lower in hospitals where 60% of the nurses had bachelors or higher degrees than in hospitals where only 20% of nurses did.

■ The results imply that, all else being equal, substantial decreases in mortality rates could result from increasing registered nurse staffing [. . .] the results [. . .] suggest that the focus on reducing nurse workloads is a credible approach to improving patient care. (Aiken, Clarke, Silber, & Sloane, 2003)

The Institute of Medicine's (IOM) report, *Keeping Patients Safe: Transforming the Work Environment of Nurses*, took a critical look at the working conditions for nurses in America's hospitals.

The nation's 2.2 million registered nurses (RNs), 700,000 licensed practical and vocational nurses, and 2.3 million nursing assistants constitute 54% of all health care providers. Nurses are the health professionals who interact most frequently with patients in all settings, and their actions—such as ongoing monitoring of patients' health status—are directly related to better patient outcomes. Studies show that increased infections, bleeding, and cardiac and respiratory failure are associated with inadequate numbers of nurses. Nurses also defend against medical errors. For example, a study in two hospitals found that nurses intercepted 86% of medication errors before they reached patients.

Despite the growing body of evidence that better nursing-staff levels result in safer patient care, nurses in some health care facilities may be overburdened. For instance, some hospital nurses may be assigned as many as 12 patients per shift. Available methods for achieving safer staffing levels—such as authorizing nursing staff to halt admissions to their units when staffing is inadequate for safe patient care—are not employed uniformly by either hospitals or nursing homes (IOM, 2004).

Organizational Research

Nurses have been unable to improve their workplace because they do not have enough power. Many organizations have dismissed nursing concerns and censured nurse reporters. This has reduced the nurses' willingness to keep trying to make improvements. Researchers at Harvard Business School examined these issues and came up with the following results:

> We propose that how employees respond to problems encountered on the job is a critical factor in enabling or preventing positive organizational change [. . .] Our analysis of quantitative data suggests that problem-solving behavior of frontline workers may reduce an organization's ability to detect underlying causes of recurring problems and thus take corrective action [. . .]
>
> The first author observed 22 nurses in eight different hospitals for a total of 197 hours. She made observations on all three shifts and on all days of the week [. . .] In 197 hours of observation of 22 nurses, we documented 120 problems (or approximately one every 1.6 hours of observation). Examples include the following.
> 1. Missing or incorrect information
> 2. Missing or broken equipment
> 3. Waiting for a resource
> 4. Missing or incorrect medication
>
> Missing or incorrect information, the most time consuming type of problem, included not having a Tylenol order to treat a patient's fever, looking for test results, and not being told about a patient's nausea during a change-of-shift report. (Tucker, Edmonson, & Spear, 2002)

Discover the reasons why health care organizations aren't learning from their mistakes. They are repeating the same mistakes over and over again, a most wasteful practice.

First-Order Problem Solving

When nurses encounter problems in their jobs, they have essentially two choices: solve only the immediate problem or solve the root cause. Consider the first choice, fixing only the immediate problem. This is called first-order problem solving. If a nurse runs out of a supply of towels, for example, they can be borrowed from someone else. This solves the immediate problem but does nothing to eliminate the cause. It also may create a problem for somebody else, because the department where the towels came from may then run out of towels.

Second-Order Problem Solving

Another choice in problem solving is to identify and eliminate the root cause of the problem as well. In other words, in addition to getting more towels, you find out why you ran out of towels in the first place. It is called second-order problem solving when you diagnose and alter the underlying cause of the problem to prevent recurrence and improve performance.

Why Is This Study Important

The nurses in the Harvard Business School study (Tucker, Edmonson, & Spear, 2002) used first-order problem solving most of the time. This means that their problems were likely to recur, because the root cause was never eliminated.

The Harvard study indicates that work environment is a critical factor in the success of clinical nurses. Organizations are failing to improve because nurses are unable to use second-order problem solving. Nurses have to face the same problems happening over and over again without much chance to intervene. It's no wonder that nurses burn out.

According to the study, health care work environments actually fostered first-order problem solving. The study found that there are three specific aspects of work environments that prevent nurses from engaging in second-order problem solving:

- Nurses have too little time to resolve the problems.
- They lack effective communication channels with people who can help.
- They have lower status relative to doctors and administrators. (All from Tucker, Edmonson, & Spear, 2002.)

I have seen managers, just like clinical nurses, who often use first-order problem solving. They try to solve staffing problems with higher salaries, sign-on bonuses, or other short-term strategies. Many health care organizations are just like the nurse who borrowed the towels and never learned why there was a shortage. Organizations poach nurses from others, without using second-order problem solving to diagnose the underlying cause of why their nurses left.

The good news is that these environmental factors are within our control and can be changed. Change may not come easily, but it is easier than enticing disenfranchised nurses to return to what has become an unsatisfactory work environment.

Implications About Safety and Quality

The towel example was a minor problem. However, the Harvard study (Tucker, Edmonson, & Spear, 2002) also uncovered the potential for larger mistakes. For example, during the study, an obstetrics nurse had a consistent problem: she found that infant security tags had fallen off on several occasions. Because the purpose of those security tags is to prevent infant abduction, the potential consequences were serious.

Ideas for Change

- Encourage nurses to use second-order problem solving to find the root causes of the problems.
- If you are the manager, be a good role model.
- If you are a clinical nurse, keep track of recurring problems and provide the necessary feedback for your organization.

A general rule of thumb for change is to address psychological, organizational, and institutional factors together.

Financial Research

The nursing shortage has resulted in a vicious cycle of cost escalation because nurse turnover includes many hidden costs. For example, organizations must spend money on advertising, interviewing, and training new staff. They may need to budget for premium pay in order to staff their facility during transition periods. New staff members are usually less productive at first, and this also costs money.

Consider the following cost estimates of nurse turnover from the Nursing Executive Center:

Typically, the accounting cost of nurse turnover per nurse is $10,800. However, that number only represents 24% of the real cost. The hidden costs—productivity costs that represent 76% of the true costs—raise the total turnover figure to $42,000.

The number is higher for specialty nurses. Here the typical accounting figure of nurse turnover for specialty nurses is $11,520. Adding the hidden costs makes the total cost for specialty-nurse turnover $64,000.

A 500-bed hospital can save $800,000 per year if administrators reduce nurse turnover from 13% a year to 10% a year, a mere 3%. (Assumptions: 500-bed hospital; 500 full-time equivalent [FTE] RNs; composition of turnover: 60% medical/surgical RNs, 40% specialty RNs) (Nursing Executive Center, 2000).

The Staffing Mix

A Commonwealth Fund study, *Is There a Business Case for Quality?* (Needleman, Buerhaus, Steward, et al., 2006), examined the safety and financial outcomes of various nurse-staffing mixes. Three staffing mixes were studied:

1.   Raising the proportion of RNs without changing the number of licensed hours.
2.   Raising the number of licensed hours without changing the proportions of RNs.
3.   Raising both the proportion of RNs and the licensed hours.

The net costs or savings (in millions) and the actual number of avoided deaths were as follows:

Strategy 1: Savings of $ 1,821 (0.5% savings) with 4,997 deaths avoided.

Strategy 2: Increased costs of $3,240 (0.8% higher costs) with 1,801 deaths avoided.

Strategy 3: Increased costs of $1,558 (0.4% higher costs) with 6,654 deaths avoided. (Needleman, Buerhaus, Steward, et al., 2006)

The research data about the nursing crisis are riveting. With so many research studies and such large patient populations studied, this research gives great validity to what nurses have been saying for many years.

Read on with a solution-oriented frame of mind. Smart Nursing provides many constructive suggestions from which to choose.

Promoting Research

TIPS FOR CLINICAL NURSES

- Keep up your computer and Web skills.
- Support new research.
- Use research for clinical decision making.
- Make use of evidence in your practice.
- Embrace change.

TIPS FOR MANAGERS

- Assist your staff to use evidence-based practice (EBP).
- Align your clinical processes with research.
- Support EBP financially.
- Network to increase use of EBP.
- Use research from other industries to learn new management practices.

TIPS FOR EDUCATORS

- Be a lifelong learner.
- Maintain your clinical skills.
- Teach about role change.
- Teach EBP with case studies.
- Perform your own research.

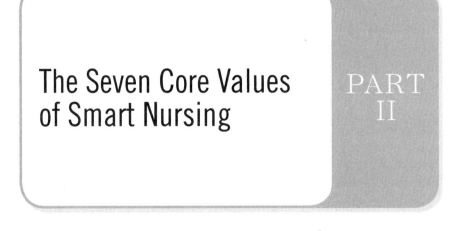

The Seven Core Values of Smart Nursing

PART II

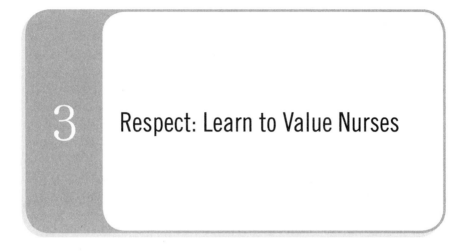

3   Respect: Learn to Value Nurses

It is part of the healthy instinctual psyche to have deep reactions to disrespect.
—*Clarissa Pinkola Estes*

Many physicians and managers have become respectful of nurses. Consider these examples:

- A physician collaborates with nurses, and together they tirelessly respond to the needs of a critically injured patient.
- A nurse, contacting a physician-on-call about her concern for a patient, receives a timely and appreciative return call.
- A physician reviews the assessments of an observant nurse and modifies the patient's treatment plan.
- A manager warmly expresses sincere gratitude to her hardworking nursing staff.
- A physician builds a warm working relationship with the nursing staff.

BEST PRACTICE: SPEED COLLABORATION

Kristin L. Gillen, MSN, RN, Director of Nursing Renown Health, Reno, NV

Renown Health, in Reno, Nevada, wanted to improve nurse physician collaboration and ultimately improve patient outcomes. We started holding biannual nurse and physician retreats to work on communication and problem-solving issues.

At the last retreat, we created an activity called "speed collaboration," based on the concept of speed dating. This provided nurses and physicians with opportunities to connect on both personal and professional levels. When presenting the study results in the fall of 2007, we wanted an open discussion, so we created an educational program with a panel of physician leaders.

Evidence

This was an evidence-based activity. We conducted research using the Jefferson Scale of Attitudes Toward Physician-Nurse Collaboration (Hojat & Herman, 1985) to examine the current attitudes toward nurse and physician collaboration. This study showed that nurses have higher positive attitudes toward collaboration overall and that shared education could potentially improve nurse and physician collaboration. We found research showing that nurse satisfaction improved when nurses worked in an environment that supported effective nurse and physician collaboration (Scott, Sochalski & Aiken, 1999).

A committee of managers and staff nurses planned and executed the retreat. At Renown Health, we continually look for opportunities to improve nurse and physician relationships, and we believe that using research is the best way to foster collaboration.

But imagine if you were a nurse in the following situations:

- You enforce a hospital-wide safety protocol and receive irate responses from physicians who feel inconvenienced.
- You report a negative response to a physician's prescribed treatment and find yourself on the receiving end of his wrath.

- You have an excellent work record but have been targeted for disrespect by your manager's ill temper.
- You are working near a highly stressed physician who takes her irritability out on you.
- You make several suggestions to solve a patient safety problem, only to be ignored by your manager. After a patient is injured, action is finally taken.
- You ask to "read-back" a physician's order to reduce medical errors, but the physician refuses to listen.

If you were the nurse in these situations, wouldn't you feel resentful? Physicians and managers who exhibit this kind of behavior are small in number, but their influence is widespread. Their actions are damaging, and they discount nurses' valuable contributions.

Eliminating Disruptive Behavior

In July 2008, the Joint Commission issued a new directive: *Behaviors that undermine a culture of safety.* This directive describes behaviors that undermine a culture of safety and lists the requirements that will become effective in January 2009.

Some of the following issues are discussed in the directive:

- Safety and quality of patient care are dependent on teamwork, communication, and a collaborative work environment.
- Disruptive behavior is not gender specific and can occur among or between groups of physicians, nurses, and other groups of health care professionals.
- Studies link patient complaints about unprofessional, disruptive behaviors and increased risk of patients bringing malpractice suits.

Effective January 1, 2009, the Joint Commission has a new leadership standard (LD.03.01.01) that recommends establishment of the following:

1. A code of conduct that defines acceptable and disruptive and inappropriate behaviors (required)
2. Process for managing disruptive and inappropriate behaviors (required)
3. Additional suggested actions, including education, reinforcement of model behaviors, establishing policies that address Zero

Tolerance, addressing issues such as fear of intimidation or retribution, and providing skills-based training, accountability, and coaching for all leaders and managers in relationship building and collaborative practice.

The need for respectful interdisciplinary relationships is addressed by the American Nurse Credentialing Center (ANCC) Magnet Force number 13: "Collaborative working relationships within and among the disciplines are valued. Mutual respect is based on the premise that all members of the health care team make essential and meaningful contributions in the achievement of clinical outcomes. Conflict management strategies should be in place and used effectively, when indicated" (ANCC, Forces of magnetism).

Applying Smart Nursing core values and adopting the guiding principles of Smart Health Care Management can help organizations apply the new Joint Commision recommendations and the ANCC Magnet Force number 13.

Other sources of disrespectful behavior come from nursing peers. Nurses who undermine others, particularly new nurses, engage in an adolescent-style interaction, resulting in petty jealousies that drive other nurses from the industry. This behavior undermines patient care, safety, and quality. The health of nurses declines when nurses are bullied. Nurses, managers, and physicians must work together to rise above this challenge.

Negative cultures prevent consumers from receiving full value for their health care dollar. Losses in nurse productivity represent a significant amount of money that could be used to add value to patient care.

Fear, miscommunication, and lack of collaboration are all root causes of medical errors such as those shown in the following examples:

- A medication dose doesn't make sense, but the nurse avoids calling for clarification because the physician has a history of angry responses.
- The operating-room staff fail to communicate the sponge count accurately. When the patient fails to heal, an X-ray reveals that a sponge had been left in the body.
- A staff member hesitates to ask for lifting help. The negative environment has conditioned him or her that asking for help is unacceptable. Both the patient and the staff member are injured by the resulting patient fall.

Disrespectful behavior toward nurses results in medical errors, chaos, and a generalized decline in quality of care.

Although organizations, managers, and physicians usually use respectful words when describing nurses, their actions often reveal the opposite. Nurses have endured censure when they have complained about management or physician directives. Prior to the current crisis, many managers summarily dismissed outspoken nurses and sought to hire more submissive ones.

A presentation called "The Color of Fear" (available at stirfryseminars.com) was a three-part seminar addressing the nature of racism. The course features a video in which minority males discuss their personal experiences with racism. I responded to the discussion in ways that puzzled me. I identified strongly with the men's feelings and asked, "Why do I, a white American female, feel so much like the minority men in the video?" The minister leading the course, familiar with the experiences of nurses working in negative cultures, replied, "It's because oppression feels the same, no matter what the cause."

Oppression feels the same, no matter what the cause.

The oppression of nurses darkens health care. As a nurse, I struggle to respond to that oppression. People often react to negativity, unthinkingly, with more negativity, but that response achieves little. Therefore, I have attempted to respond to health care negativity with many positive solutions.

Gary Zukav, in his book *The Seat of the Soul*, likens evil to darkness. He said that we can't eliminate darkness with more darkness. We can only remove it with light. Similarly, we can only replace disrespect by developing respect (Zukav, 1990).

Employers who treat nurses with disrespect have eroded nurse self-respect. They delude themselves when they expect nurses to be productive if they are working under such conditions. What they don't realize is that the most accurate and productive nurses are the ones with the most self-respect.

Researchers at Wharton, interested in whether respectful or disrespect treatment influenced employee burnout, came to the following conclusions:

- Organizational respect influences burnout above and beyond the effects of job demands and negative affectivity.

- The impact of organizational respect on burnout is felt most strongly when job autonomy is low.
- The respect with which an organization treats its employees is a pervasive organizational-level phenomenon.
- One's perception of respect and disrespect are not only based on how one views one's own treatment, but also by how others are treated. (Barsade & Ramarajan, 2006)

Consider how this study applies to the nursing shortage:

- Nurses are affected by the degree of respect exhibited in the workplace.
- Nurses without autonomy are more affected by a lack of respect and are more likely to experience burnout.
- The presence or absence of respect usually affects every nurse within the organization.
- When nurses see others being treated with disrespect, they are more likely to experience burnout.

One reason that nurses without autonomy are more likely to experience burnout is as a result of the greater amount of stress that people feel when they cannot influence their situation. Autonomous nurses, who might at least have a chance to improve their situation, experience less stress and are less likely to burn out.

Some progressive managers are actively curbing nurse disrespect with sanctions. A few have even gone as far as filing complaints to the medical board. As a result, some physicians have had to change their behavior or lose their medical licenses. But all too frequently, the abusive behavior continues.

Three no-cost ways to counteract the burnout that the Wharton study suggests are the following:

- Treat every employee at every level with respect.
- Support employee autonomy.
- Create, support, and model a culture of respect throughout the organization.

Respect is related to power and control issues. Unfortunately, many respectful physicians and managers consistently look the other way and do not police their own. This reluctance to intervene turns many health care centers into epicenters of harm instead of centers for healing. As a result, many ill-treated but caring nurses have left health care for other employment.

In the book *The Real Wealth of Nations* (2007), two power options for systems and societies are contrasted:

1. A domination system in which there are only two choices: dominating or being dominated.
2. A partnership system that supports mutually respectful relations. Hierarchies are still needed to get things done, but these are hierarchies of actualization rather than hierarchies of domination. Accountability and respect flow both ways rather than just from the bottom up (Eisler, 2007).

Although no society or system makes use only of one or the other power system, those that apply partnership model principles form more caring and respectful societies or systems. The partnership model would be a helpful guide in making our health care system more respectful of both staff and patients.

Trust is necessary for patient safety, nurse recruitment, and teamwork. When nurses trust physicians and managers, they feel comfortable being autonomous. This enables them to be fully engaged in caring for patients—without having to waste time wondering whether they will be supported—thus raising nurse productivity the right way.

How do you build trust? You build trust by respecting yourself and others. You build it by being a role model, by courteous communication, and by sensitivity to the needs of others. Staff members pay attention when you seek them out and ask for their input. Nurses trust you when you consistently make decisions according to what is right rather than what is easy.

Abraham Maslow developed his hierarchy of needs in *Motivation and Personality* (Maslow, 1954). Nurses and other health care professionals have used this philosophy to understand patient behavior, but they don't usually think of it as affecting themselves. Take a fresh look at Maslow's hierarchy to understand the nursing crisis. We use this hierarchy in patient care to understand patients. Those who struggle to obtain their basic needs for food and shelter may not be able to concentrate on higher-level needs such as education.

What happens when we apply Maslow's ideas to nursing? A nurse who transfers patients with too few staff might have to contend with a serious back injury. This is a violation of a nurse's basic physical needs. Or what about nurse Jones, who arrives at work to find that only three licensed staff are working instead of the usual five. Nurse Jones is scared and angry. She is scared that she will miss treatable complications or make a serious medical error. She is angry because so many previous nurses have resigned because of multiple understaffing situations. Management has violated nurse Jones's basic need for safety and security. Are you ignoring Maslow's hierarchy of needs relative to nurses?

Types of Disrespect

Lack of respect for nurses includes both active and passive types. Active disrespectful behavior includes blatant verbal abuse. For example, a physician whose patient is in physical decline yells at the patient's nurse. The nurse may even have been the astute one—the one to notice the patient's symptoms first. But the nurse, the one without power, can be targeted for disrespect, and he or she has little recourse.

Passive disrespectful behavior involves disregarding nurse input. Like physicians, experienced nurses are very skilled at noticing when patients start going into physical decline. You might call it intuition. Their intuition has been honed by many years of experience and education. During nursing seminars, I often ask nurses if they have picked up on important patient problems early by using their intuition. Most of the hands immediately go up, and the nurses are able to cite many examples of the ways that their intuition has benefited patients. The best physicians pay attention to nurses because astute nurses add value to their medical interventions.

Reasonable assignments demonstrate that managers care about the long-term physical and emotional health of their staff; tired nurses cannot respond well to patient needs. Maximizing both the nursing effectiveness and the resulting quality care is what determines your reputation and whether you will be profitable.

Promoting Respect of Nurses

TIPS FOR CLINICAL NURSES

- Maintain your self-respect.
- Build alliances.
- Learn to negotiate well.
- Support respectful behavior.
- Reduce negativity over past events.

TIPS FOR MANAGERS

- Deal promptly with issues of disrespect.
- Build trust.
- Show appreciation.
- Do what's right, not just what's easy.
- Support your nurses.

TIPS FOR EDUCATORS

- Discuss the respect issue.
- Teach assertiveness skills.
- Be a role model.
- Discuss respect with clinical staff.
- Role-play potential challenging situations.

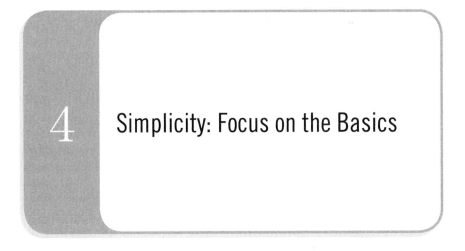

4   Simplicity: Focus on the Basics

Waste thrives on complexity; effectiveness requires simplicity.   —*Richard Koch*

Simplicity involves rethinking our priorities and returning to basic values of trust, respect, and common sense. It is different from over-simplification, which is the desire to find simple solutions for complex problems.

Patient safety should be our most important goal. Some of the keys to patient safety are hiring the right people, hiring enough of them, and providing an environment where they can use their full professional capacity. Whom should you hire? Hire nurses who are able to think critically, have strong personal and professional values, and exhibit excellent interpersonal skills. Then give them the freedom to use their professional judgment and determine the best way to satisfy your clients.

Health care is not the only industry that has stifled autonomous professionals. Analysis of NASA's *Challenger* tragedy has revealed that professional engineers, who were the most knowledgeable about O-rings, had warned NASA about O-ring failures at low temperatures, but they were ignored. Nurses have been warning their organizations about unsafe staffing for years, but they too have been ignored.

Health care complexity causes medical errors, contributes to the nursing shortage, and reduces productivity. Simplification enables staff to remove this obstacle. William Jessee describes the dangers of complexity this way:

> Frustration with the administrative complexity of the U.S. healthcare system has reached a fever pitch. Patients, payers, physicians and policy-makers agree on at least one thing: the complexity costs big money but does nothing to improve patient care. . . [money] and medical opportunity—is wasted in a system that bases a bewildering array of clinical guidelines, diseases management protocols, specialist referral requirements, drug formularies and other aspects of patient care on which health plan the patient is enrolled in, rather than on scientific evidence of what works best . . . the current duplicative, costly redundant system is harming the nation's health. It's time for a change. (Jessee, 2003)

Complexity is unsafe because excessively detailed safety standards rarely match patient situations. The best way to use your policies is to rely on the judgment of professional nurses as they implement them in a thoughtful way. Our increasingly diverse patient population will continue to raise the need for professionals who know how to think critically.

Lean Management in Health Care

Smart Nursing core values and guiding principles of health care management complement "lean" management strategies that have important applications to health care. In his book, *The 80/20 Principle, The Secret of Achieving More with Less*, Richard Koch (1998) addresses "cost reduction through simplicity" this way:

> There is a natural tendency for business, like life in general, to become overly complex . . . . [Organizations] do not focus on what they should be doing. They should be adding value to their customers and potential customers . . . It follows that any organization always has great potential for cost reduction and for delivering better value to customers: by simplifying what it does and by eliminating low or negative-value activities . . . Major improvements are always possible, by doing things differently and doing less. (Koch, 1998)

These remarks are based on the Pareto Principle, first identified by Italian economist Vilfredo Pareto (1848–1923). This principle demonstrates that 20% of one's resources account for approximately 80% of the results. Sales managers use this idea to identify their top sales people, whereby 20% of their sales force is usually responsible for 80% of the sales. (You can even apply it humorously in our weight-conscious society by saying, "Twenty percent of our food is responsible for 80% of our weight gain.") Working smarter, not harder, is another way to summarize the Pareto Principle.

This idea can be used to set priorities. For example, Elizabeth, a nurse manager, might ask herself, "Which 20% of my actions will produce 80% of my desired results?" The following five choices might enable Elizabeth to achieve her goals of excellence more efficiently:

- Spending time solving the root causes of problems
- Hiring competent staff
- Responding to patient and staffing issues promptly
- Consistently practicing ethical behaviors
- Focusing on patient needs

Practicing these principles enables organizations to focus on the future. Cindy, a clinical nurse, might ask herself the same questions that Elizabeth asked. How can she maximize her time to achieve the best results?

- Use her intuition about patient symptoms and intervene early.
- Limit her work hours so that she is able to feel well rested.
- Use a flexible approach when responding to patient requests.
- Communicate with compassion and respect.
- Collaborate with others to raise productivity without fatigue.

The Pareto Principle is similar to the concept of leverage. A lever is a simple machine that allows you to multiply your results. If you are a gardener, you might use a crowbar as a lever to lift a heavy rock out of your garden. Without the crowbar, the rock would have been too heavy.

When you use the Pareto Principle you can expect the following outcomes:

- Increased flexibility results in customized medical care.
- Faster decision making highlights the value of autonomous nurses.
- High levels of employee and client satisfaction build organizational success.

Smart Nursing core values and guiding principles enable you to leverage scarce health care resources and to do more with less. You may have to make some trade-offs (slay some sacred cows?). Are you willing to make the following trade-offs?

- Give up micromanagement and choose delegation.
- Give up instant gratification and choose long-term results.
- Give up what is easy and choose what is right.
- Give up control and choose staff autonomy.
- Give up rigidity and choose flexibility.
- Give up talking and choose listening.
- Give up judging and choose empathy.
- Give up victimization and choose accountability.
- Give up ego and choose teamwork.
- Give up punishment and choose education.
- Give up coercion and choose negotiation.
- Give up the status quo and choose innovation.
- Give up arrogance and choose humility.
- Give up carelessness and choose safety.
- Give up stress and choose humor.

The next step of simplification is to focus on what is most important to you. The following are some ideas for projects:

- Put less time pressure on nurses, in order to decrease their need to rush through patient care.
- Promote autonomy and assertive communication.
- Plan informal social events.
- Transform waste into something on your wish list; for example, save $5,000 on wasted supplies and use it for unit education.
- Reduce duplication and increase direct time with patients.

Become a Boundaryless Organization

Organizations need structure to function in an organized manner, but health care organizations often allow boundaries to wall themselves off from their staff. One of our most destructive boundaries is the authoritarian boundary. Health care's command and control atmosphere has blocked communication, innovation, and relationships. We have paid a high price: medical errors, high staff turnover, and financial insolvency.

These boundaries have sabotaged staff's pride in a job well done. We need nurse pride, licensed nurse aide/certified nurse aide (LNA/CNA) pride, and housekeeping pride. Every health care staff member is equally important. Do you realize that clinical staff are often judged by how clean you keep your facility? This is yet another example of the importance of valuing every employee, no matter what his or her responsibilities are.

Boundaryless organizations represent simplicity because they use common sense as a guide to making decisions. Jack Welch, in his book *Jack: Straight from the Gut* (2001), shared this experience about removing boundaries. His executives needed computer coaching; Generation X employees, who grew up with computers, were the experts. Welch authorized the Generation Xers to become computer coaches for his executives, despite the fact that the executives had higher status positions. He used common sense and matched up those who knew a skill with those who needed to know it—simplicity in action.

Researchers have found that eliminating bureaucracy has been a driver of the most highly productive companies, worldwide. "This place works because of the collaborative efforts of everyone. We have no time or place for self-absorbed egotists" (Jennings, 2002). Jennings goes on to say that "bureaucracies waste money, show disrespect for workers, destroy competitive spirits, and don't fit the goal of simple (Jennings, 2002).

Nurses are clinical experts who are eager to share their knowledge, and they are seeking listeners who are just as eager to use that expertise to benefit patients.

How to Simplify

1. Make time to reflect.

    Time for reflection enables staff to work smarter, not just harder. Reflection during quiet times enables new ideas to surface from the deeper, problem-solving areas of the brain.
2. Reduce duplication.

    Many times, nurses must document the same information in four or five places. Sometimes this repetition is necessary for legal reasons, but much of it can be eliminated.
3. Adopt zero-based planning.

    Years ago, there was a popular concept called zero-based budgeting. The idea behind it was to start writing a budget with a zero in every column and then justify the necessity of each entry. This practice eliminated grandfathering everything in from the prior year, without acknowledging its necessity. We can do the same; justify every bit of complexity to ensure its necessity.

4. Keep your mind open to new ideas.

One nurse in the 1980s took a trip to Disney World and was impressed by their customer service. She asked to use a modified version at work, but management declined. Now, 20 years later, health care organizations are eager to learn about Disney's version of customer service.

Ask yourself this question: What ideas are we now rejecting that will become the gold standard for 2020? It's time to simplify, simplify, simplify.

Promoting Simplicity

TIPS FOR CLINICAL NURSES

- Pay attention to unnecessary complexity.
- Look for simpler ways to do your work.
- Praise success stories of simplicity.
- Take time to reflect.
- Share knowledge with others.

TIPS FOR MANAGERS

- Give your nurses autonomy to simplify problem solving.
- Seek out root causes of problems.
- Talk with managers from other industries.
- Use leverage.
- Walk your talk.

TIPS FOR EDUCATORS

- Add decision-making strategies to your curriculum.
- Teach simplification.
- Discuss occupational barriers.
- Simplify your curriculum.
- Encourage students to reflect on their work.

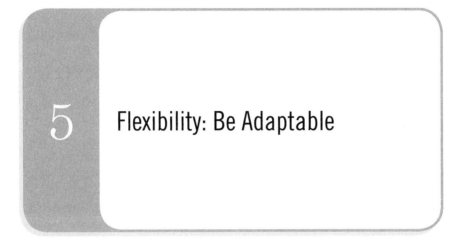

5 Flexibility: Be Adaptable

It is not necessary to change. Survival is not mandatory.
—*W. Edwards Deming*

Health care consumers need flexibility because our diverse society requires the critical thinking skills of autonomous caregivers.

As mentioned in the introduction, both nursing process and Smart Nursing strategies are based on general systems theory, which focuses on the wholeness of a situation. Our organizations are not linear; they are complex adaptive systems. Peter Senge uses the analogy of weather to describe the behavior of complex adaptive systems:

> A cloud masses, the sky darkens, leaves twist upward, and we know it will rain. We also know that after the storm, the runoff will feed into groundwater miles away, and the sky will grow clear by tomorrow. These events are distant in time and space, and yet they are all connected with the same pattern. Each has an influence on the rest, an influence that is usually hidden from view. You can only understand the system of the rainstorm by contemplating the whole. (Senge, 1990)

Business and other human systems are bound by invisible fabrics of interrelated actions, which often take years to play out. When we focus on isolated parts of the health care system, we don't realize that we only have a snapshot of the problem. We wonder why our deepest problems never get solved. Systems thinking is a conceptual framework, a body of knowledge and group of tools developed over the past fifty years, that provides the know-how to improve our systems (Senge, 1990).

Critical Thinking Skills

Critical thinking implies that an organization has the flexibility to change as circumstances do. Managers frequently lament that they need nurses who can think critically, yet they fail to realize that critical thinkers need an environment that is based on freedom and autonomy. When nurses hesitate to make the independent decisions related to critical thinking, it's because they have been reprimanded for doing so in the past. They have learned to hedge when faced with choices because their experiences have taught them that hedging is safer than taking a stand. This ingrained habit is difficult to break. The best way to slowly change this habit is to build trust by giving your nurses consistent support.

Policies are black and white, but patient needs come in shades of gray. That is why we need competent professionals. We need nurses with good judgment and critical thinking skills to apply organizational policies to patient needs in a way that makes sense for patients. Health care employees are more important than ever because their collective knowledge comprises the intellectual capital of their organization.

Flexibility reduces waste because patients receive only the services that they actually need. A less expensive alternative, excluded by rigid policies, often is more satisfactory to patients. For instance, a patient who is entitled to spend time in a rehabilitation center may prefer less expensive home care.

How Managers Can Encourage The Critical Thinking of Clinical Nurses

- Make your nurses feel safe when being decisive. Always support them. Delegate decision-making authority.
- Coach your nurses so that they can tweak their decision-making skills. Sit down with staff members periodically, review their recent decisions, and guide them in becoming even better decision makers.

- Give positive feedback so that clinical staff want to continue being decisive. Clinical nurses who are sure of their manager's support outperform other nurses.
- Celebrate your successes. Find ways to reward nurses who make good decisions.

WHY DON'T NURSES SAY YES TO PATIENTS MORE OFTEN?

Nurses feel safe when they can say, "I followed policy to the letter," even if patient needs remain unmet.

How Clinical Nurses Can Cultivate Critical Thinking Skills

- Ask yourself the following question: Is this patient request illegal, unethical, or harmful? If not, find a way to fulfill most requests to a patient's satisfaction.
- Put yourself in the patient's place. Ask yourself what is motivating this patient. Why is this issue important to the patient?
- Instead of saying no, find a way to say yes. When patients ask for something, listen fully, and give them what they want, if at all possible.
- Use your creativity. Innovate and start new patient-satisfaction trends.

Rigidity Is Expensive

Rigidity wastes nursing time, because rigid protocols are hurdles for nurses to clear before they can focus on patient needs. Autonomous nurses who satisfy patients' needs with flexibility save time and raise patient satisfaction. Multiply these small segments of time saved by the number of nurses in your facility and then by their salary. The financial savings add up quickly.

Rigidity interferes with patient satisfaction because patients dislike waiting to have their needs met unless there is a good reason for the delay. Rigidity blocks patient safety because it prevents nurses from quickly sizing up the situation and taking action to solve urgent problems.

Bureaucracy

Bureaucracy sabotages individual effort. Many health care systems merged during the last 10 years in order to survive, forming integrated networks composed of hospitals, physician practices, medical specialty groups, home care companies, and satellite hospitals. This strategy has been the opposite of what others have done: become smaller, decentralized, and leaner. Be more flexible and able to respond quickly to shifting market demand. It is more important than ever for nurses to be autonomous and able to make patient care decisions at the patient level.

Consider the following two scenarios and decide which staff member you would prefer if you were Mr. Jones.

FIRST SCENARIO

Mr. Jones, a patient who is 100 pounds overweight, has been put on a 1,000-calorie weight-reduction diet during his stay at a long-term-care facility until his leg ulcers heal. He receives half a hamburger, a few vegetables and pieces of fruit, and black coffee for lunch. Mr. Jones's resentment about his dietary restrictions and lack of dietary control builds every day. Will this dietary regime provide any long-term benefit for Mr. Jones? Hardly. Mr. Jones will probably eat even more when his stay in the long-term facility is over.

SECOND SCENARIO

Nurse Smith understands how to make a real difference with Mr. Jones. She asks his doctor to order a regular diet, enabling him to make his own food choices. Along with the dietician, she works with Mr. Jones to learn how to make better food choices. She asks the food service to provide Mr. Jones with high-bulk, low-calorie foods, such as stir-fries and vegetable soups. She reminds him how weight reduction can improve his quality of life and enable him to return to his hobby of fly-fishing. Motivation, flexibility, and patient involvement make a big difference to Mr. Jones, who continues to lose weight gradually after discharge.

In the first scenario, the staff required Mr. Jones to follow a rigid, senseless plan. In the second, nurse Smith thought critically and used a flexible approach. Although Mr. Jones was not able to lose a dramatic amount of weight immediately, nurse Smith's thoughtful intervention started him on the road to healthier living.

Flexibility Strengthens Medical Ethics

Organizations often think that rigidity is the best way to provide ethical care, but that is not so. Read what Marvin T. Brown says in his book *Working Ethics*:

> People . . . interested in ethics will understand the differences between an ethics of rules, which attempts to control behavior, and an ethics of decision making, which empowers people and organizations. (Brown, 1990)

Staff empowerment is again considered to be vital. Consider how this concept can be applied to the nursing crisis. A charge nurse discovers that a patient is in physical decline. She reports the patient's deteriorating condition to the physician, who fails to grasp the severity of the situation. The charge nurse, who takes her ethical responsibility seriously, confers with the supervisor. Supervisors generally choose one of two options. They do what is easy. If they fear offending the physician, they play it safe and fail to act, which leaves nurses without any support while advocating for patients. Or supervisors do what is right. Great supervisors choose the second option and do what is right despite potential criticism and political risk. Consider this example of doing what is right:

> After a supervisor conferred with a charge nurse about a patient's deteriorating condition, she called the physician back herself. Although the physician lived 30 minutes away and the time was 10:30 at night, he arrived at the hospital to examine the patient within 45 minutes.

This illustrates how the ethics of decision making empowers people. The supervisor, as an empowered manager, intervened appropriately to promote the patient's best interest.

Consider the following example about the benefits of flexibility for patient care as reported by W. Mitchell, a paraplegic patient who was undergoing rehabilitation. He had already recovered from severe burns from a prior accident.

> I had to fight mighty battles for privileges that are taken for granted in the real world . . . For example, there was the battle of the telephone system. When this second accident had occurred, I was quite a successful businessman with interests and investments all across the nation. On a normal day, I made perhaps thirty telephone calls, and I had no intention

of changing that. The insistence on rest and quiet in hospitals is often just an invitation for the patient to worry about his awful fate. I chose to get on with my life.

The hospital's telephone system required every call to go through an overworked operator, and it shut down completely at 8 p.m. It was adequate for chatting with one's wife about how the kids are doing in school. It was a disaster for someone with needs like mine . . . I actually became the first patient in the history of that hospital to have a private, outside line strung into my room at my request, and at my expense, of course. (Mitchell, 1997)

Mitchell's long-term goal was probably to achieve maximum physical and mental functioning. Following hospital policy and denying Mitchell the phone line sabotaged this goal and was the opposite of his plan. Was Mitchell's request illegal, unethical, or harmful? No! Consider how a lack of critical thinking would have interfered with Mitchell's recovery had he not insisted on having his needs met:

- It would have reduced his rehabilitation potential.
- It would have disrupted his relationship with the treatment team.
- It would have compromised his ability to function as a successful businessman.

Times Are Changing

Complex health conditions demand flexibility. Our increasingly diverse population and 24-7 culture has created an expectation of flexibility. Our nursing role will become more advisory and less regulatory in the future. The Internet has enabled patients to collect abundant data, but it has not helped them interpret the information. Nurses can assist patients to use information from the Web constructively, in order to make smart health care decisions.

Escalating medical error rates often influence staff to become even more rigid.

> The rigidity of the ethics of rules has become another root cause for errors, because it leaves no room for professional judgment as in the ethics of decision making.

Clinical Nurses and Staffing Flexibility

Sally arrives for work at 11:00 p.m. She hears that the supervisor has been unable to replace two nurses who have "called out." Sally wishes that she had called out too; then she would have been able to avoid this problem. Sally knows that she will be expected to manage a much larger assignment. But she also knows that the patient acuity is very high and that, if she accepts too heavy an assignment, she risks making serious errors.

Although Sally wants to be a team player, she knows that this kind of situation happens frequently, resulting in a vicious cycle of nurses burning out and seeking other careers. Sally knows that if she is too flexible, management will not solve the root causes of the staffing problems, and she will end up enabling a dysfunctional system to continue.

A Manager's Perspective on Staffing Flexibility

Your job as a manager involves scheduling adequate staff and ensuring patient safety. Because short patient stays result in large numbers of unplanned admissions and discharges, unit acuity can shift dramatically hour by hour. It makes no sense to be overstaffed on one unit and understaffed on another. But the nurses complain every time you ask them to float to another unit. You think to yourself, "Can't the nurses be a little more flexible?"

The Root Causes of Inflexibility

Obsolete Power Structures

Many health care organizations have remained autocratic, and their centralized command and control structures are slow and ineffective. Obsolete power structures cause organizations to sacrifice three important goals: customer satisfaction, profitability, and productivity.

Exploitation

As members of one of the helping professions, many nurses report that their profession has deepened their generous nature. As a result, they often feel obliged to work extra hours so that their colleagues are supported and patient care doesn't suffer They feel substantial guilt, thinking that patient needs will go unmet if they don't volunteer to work extra shifts.

A certain amount of generosity is commendable, but nurses burn out when managers constantly ask them to relinquish their free time to fill staffing holes. With fewer nurses, the vicious burnout cycle goes round and round. Consider the following example of the exploitation of nurses' generous natures:

A nurse answered an ad from a staffing agency and arranged an interview. When the nurse arrived, she introduced herself. No one said hello; they didn't introduce themselves; they didn't even describe the work. They gave her an application, showed her where to sit, and asked her to fill out the application.

Naturally, the nurse asked a few questions. First, she asked about the nature of the work and then about the salary. When they quoted the salary, it was a rate of pay only 50% of the usual rate for the area. When she questioned the manager about the low salary, he replied, "Well, the nurses do it to help out." It was an egregious exploitation of nurses' generous natures.

Discomfort With Ambiguity

Our environment is becoming more ambiguous, and nurses need greater self-confidence in their ability to make smart choices. Because everyone needs to pick his or her battles in life, nurses need to decide whether a particular work problem is important enough to take a stand or if they should just go with the flow. If they decide to take a stand, they need to choose the best way to be effective. And they need to decide if they are willing to accept the potential consequences.

Fear of The Unknown

Change feels uncomfortable at first, and people are more likely to make a few errors when they learn new skills. For example, learning to write for publication is often slow in the beginning but rapidly accelerates with regular practice. Many times, comfort zones eventually become more like jails when people consistently refuse to accept new opportunities. Because health care changes rapidly, nurses who refuse to change may find their job opportunities reduced as a result of obsolete skills.

Peer Pressure

People need support in order to work in challenging environments. If support for flexibility and critical thinking is absent, nurses become cynical and rigid, with a reduced sense of trust. They band together and close their minds to new management initiatives.

Solutions

Create a Culture of Appreciation

Low morale is inevitable when nurses are continuously understaffed, are working in disrespectful environments, or are censured for speaking up. Solutions to these issues are challenging, but resolution is definitely management's responsibility. Managers can show their appreciation by their actions:

- Be trustworthy.
- Promote open communication.
- Maintain a respectful workplace.
- Say thank you.
- Wheel and deal. For instance, say, "If you work on Thursday, I will give you the 3-day weekend off." Or offer time off during less busy times.

SAMPLE CONVERSATION

Manager: Because we have a high census tonight, we need an extra nurse tomorrow. I know it is your day off, but is there any chance that you could work tomorrow and take a different day off? I would really appreciate it.

Clinical nurse: Well, I have Saturday off, and taking Friday off too would be nice. I can do it.

Manager: OK. Sharon wants to work on Friday. She can take your place. Thanks for being so flexible.

Encourage a Healthy Balance Between Work and Life

A healthy balance between work and life for clinical nurses also promotes patient safety. Nurses want to have a life as well as to make a living. Retention increases when you offer nurses a challenging career that doesn't consume all of their energy. Having energetic, well-rested employees results in greater safety and higher profitability.

Offer Self-Development Opportunities

Promote an entrepreneurial attitude. Assign nurses to work on patient safety projects. Empower, coach, and support them. Everybody wins when employees become lifelong learners and increase their skills.

A Multigenerational Workforce

We now have four generations of nurses working side by side: Matures, Baby Boomers, Generation Xers, and Generation Ys. Generational differences are potential sources of conflict, but not when we value what each generation brings to the table.

The Matures (or traditionalists), born between 1900 and 1945, number about 75 million people. The Baby Boomers (1946–1964) are at 80 million. Generation Xers (1965–1980) number 46 million, and Generation Ys (or the Millennials) are at 76 million (Lancaster, 2002).

Consider what we can learn from Generation X, who are thought to have the following attributes:

- They want independence.
- They value a satisfactory balance between work and life.
- They desire self-development opportunities.

Mature generation nurses, also called the silent generation, were too silent about disrespectful behavior and the lack of autonomy. They have left a legacy of caring—but also one of powerlessness.

It is easy to see why health care cultures can be mismatches for Generation X nurses. Traditional top-down management styles discourage nurses from being independent and accountable. Frequent use of mandatory overtime prevents nurses from maintaining a healthy balance between work and life. Too often, we expect nurses to sacrifice their own needs for the good of the organization. This is another example of why quick fixes don't work. The organization will eventually lose the Generation X nurse to burnout, making the decision a very poor long-term strategy.

Nurses from the Mature and Baby Boomer generations have expertise that health care organizations need, so it is important that we retain these nurses as they age. It is also important that we understand the process by which people become experts. Expert nurses are able to size up a situation within a few seconds and know what is wrong with a patient.

How do expert nurses reach this point? (See Chapter 17 on lifelong learning to understand this "expert-building" process.) Perhaps we can replicate and accelerate the expert-building process for new nurses.

Promoting Flexibility

TIPS FOR CLINICAL NURSES

- Use common sense.
- Work toward high patient satisfaction.
- Innovate.
- Become partners with management.
- Manage stress with a sense of humor.

TIPS FOR MANAGERS

- Support staff's critical thinking.
- Be flexible yourself.
- Decrease the waste of unnecessary complexity.
- Reduce bureaucracy.
- Expect your nurses to make decisions at the patient level.

TIPS FOR EDUCATORS

- Encourage students to think for themselves.
- Talk about the power of innovation.
- Develop nurses' critical thinking skills.
- Be a flexible instructor.
- Become educated about health care economics.

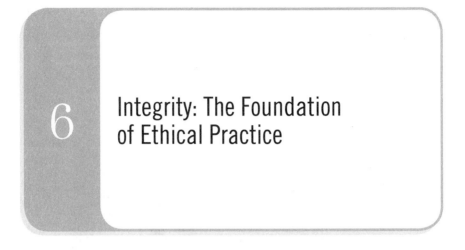

6 Integrity: The Foundation of Ethical Practice

Integrity is not just a noble idea, it's a tool for personal and corporate success.
—Gay Hendricks

Are you faced with the dilemma of maintaining your integrity while constantly adapting to change? Many times, it's hard to know what to change and what to preserve. Sometimes it takes a crisis to differentiate between those who choose honesty as a core value and others who think of integrity as merely a public relations convenience.

Integrity empowers you and is an antidote to chaos, because it increases self-respect. High self-respect creates order in your life because it is the one constant that you can depend on when everything around you is in turmoil.

Integrity has practical advantages because it saves you time and energy. In his book *The Road Less Traveled*, M. Scott Peck explains the convenience of honesty this way:

> [People] don't have to construct new lies to cover old ones. They need waste no effort covering tracks or maintaining disguises. And ultimately they find that the energy required for the self discipline of honesty is far less than the energy required for secretiveness. (Peck, 1978)

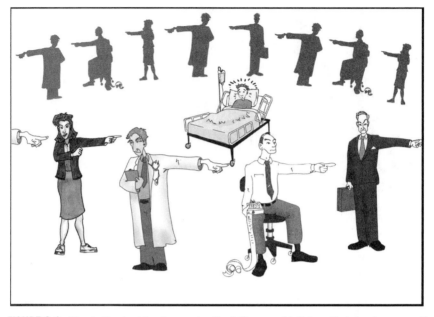

FIGURE 6.1   "Look, they're blaming each other! They wouldn't turn their backs on me if they had to wear a 'Johnnie' like I do."

For his book *The Millionaire Mind*, author Thomas J. Stanley interviewed 733 self-made millionaires and asked them to rate their most important secrets to success. Honesty was rated number one (Stanley, 2000).

Integrity is a sign of strength. Failing organizations are the ones most likely to resort to unscrupulous actions. When weak people realize that their inadequate abilities don't measure up and that they are unable to succeed by being smart enough, they try to achieve their goals with dishonesty (see Figure 6.1).

Ten Habits for Developing Integrity

1. Remain committed to integrity. Some people like the idea of integrity but discard it during tough times. Others can maintain their integrity through turbulent times. Why? They have adopted effective habits that enable them to thrive in the uncertain world where we live.

2. Pick your battles. Focus on what is important. Working within our diverse society means that others act with different styles. Without adequate understanding, these styles can seem threatening.

Learn to differentiate between differences in values and differences in style. With style differences, go with the flow. But stand firm with values conflicts. You will burn out if you allow every minor difference to upset you. Prioritize and decide which issues are most important.

3. Assess the motivations of others. If someone behaves in a questionable way, ask yourself whether inadequate education is the cause or whether there was malicious intent. Suppose someone neglected to report information to a physician. It makes a difference if the error was an oversight as a result of poor organizational skills or if the information was deliberately withheld. Each circumstance requires a different response.

4. Develop patience and persistence. Be patient and persistent with yourself as well as with others. It takes time for people to change, so you need to have a long-term approach.

5. Be specific. Clarify exactly what needs to be changed. If you want to change something about yourself, define your goal and create an action plan. If you want other people to change, ask them to summarize your request in their own words to be sure that they understand. Expect some errors at first and be willing to be a coach.

6. Use praise. Remember to praise yourself as well as others. We all enjoy approval. Even with difficult tasks, people usually respond to praise by renewing their efforts.

7. Learn multiple styles of response. Using different approaches for different people is a wise choice. Multiple styles of response enable you to choose the most appropriate one for each occasion, just as you choose different ways to dress for various occasions. Using multiple styles doesn't change your basic identity any more than changing your clothes does, and people appreciate the individual attention.

8. Use your intuition. Most people have developed intuition from their accrued knowledge and experience. This is your inner wisdom. Use it. In his book *The Confident Decision Maker*, Roger Dawson says, "Use logic as a tool, but to be a great decision maker, you must blend in the magic of intuition" (Dawson, 1993). One of Dawson's suggestions is to write down five major decisions. First, determine whether they were good or bad decisions. Then analyze whether you used mainly intuition or logic. When I did this exercise, I discovered that my best decisions

were mainly intuitive. When I use this exercise in seminars, the group is usually split 50–50. When you have enough time, it is perfectly acceptable to have an intuitive feeling about it but then put your decision on the back burner to give yourself time to reflect. As time goes on, you can determine whether your decision was a good one.

9. Cultivate a network of good people. Few people thrive in isolation; most of us need supportive people. Spend as much time as possible around other people who practice integrity. You motivate and support each other. You will have a dependable group of people to call on; it's helpful to have a reliable network already in place when new opportunities become available.

10. Welcome personal and professional growth. When you have integrity, you become real. You solidify your self-respect, which is the basic ingredient of self-confidence. It grounds you, and other people respect the consistent thread of integrity throughout all of your activities. It strengthens everything that you do.

Patient trust is very important, and caregivers need integrity if they expect to earn it. Some people try to fake integrity, but patients quickly discover the truth and discount the false messages. In contrast, patients who trust their caregivers build relationships that enable them to receive greater benefit from their treatment plans.

Multimillion-dollar deals, as well as pressure for profitability, tempt people to stray from the path of integrity. Long-term profitability disappears when companies lose their credibility by failing to value honesty.

Most health care professionals prefer working for an organization whose mission matches their personal value system. But many professional nurses receive mixed messages from their organizations, making it difficult to understand what an organization's mission really is.

A Reflection on Ethics

In his book *Working Ethics*, Marvin T. Brown advocates using ethical reflection to assist in decision making:

> The first and primary condition for ethical reflection is the organization's moral community and the moral life of its members and constituencies.

How we live with others, our environment, and ourselves constitutes our moral life [. . .] The independence of ethics comes from the act of reflection—of thinking about our moral response to situations [. . .] Ethical reflection should not be seen as some isolated activity apart from the regular process of making decisions. Instead, ethical reflection belongs within the already established decision-making processes, in dialogue with other types of methods for deciding what should be done.

For ethical reflection to be effective and to actually elicit participation, the process itself must be empowered, which in turn empowers those who engage in it. (Brown, 1990)

Suppose an organization decides to cover up a mistake. They will have to add more fabrications as time goes on. Their deceit will snowball, and they will need to spend most of their time and energy covering their tracks. Such organizations raise their risk of failure because they will have little time and energy available for positive pursuits.

Practicing Integrity in a Culture of Safety

One goal for organizations is to create safe spaces in which to set aside time to talk about patient safety.

According to Julianne Morath, in *Nursing Economics*, "Patient safety begins with fostering a blameless, yet accountable, culture . . . which values and rewards open communication and transparency. Personal and organizational honesty are not only encouraged, but expected" (Morath and Leary, 2004).

Integrity preserves staff energy and prevents future problems. The consistent practice of integrity builds staff respect, motivation, and productivity.

Promoting Integrity

TIPS FOR CLINICAL NURSES

- Be consistent.
- Pick your battles.
- Be persistent.
- Use your intuition.
- With issues of style, go with the flow. With values issues, stand fast.

TIPS FOR MANAGERS

- Use a long-term perspective.
- Praise examples of integrity.
- Hire staff with high integrity.
- Build a culture that values integrity.
- Encourage staff independence.

TIPS FOR EDUCATORS

- Include integrity in your ethics curriculum.
- Include news reports of integrity issues.
- Be honest about industry issues, to decrease reality shock for new graduates.
- Keep up your own knowledge of what is being written about integrity and ethics.
- Encourage abstract thinking.

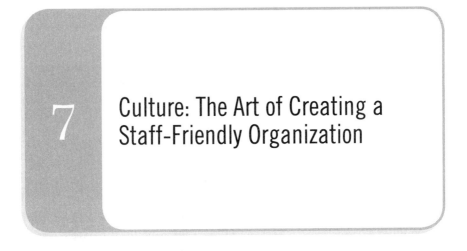

Culture: The Art of Creating a Staff-Friendly Organization

7

When you combine a culture of discipline with an ethic of entrepreneurship, you get the magical alchemy of great performance. —*Jim Collins*

Culture matters. Any group achieving long-term success—whether a work group, a family, or a professional organization—most likely has a positive culture. Consider how one work group promotes enthusiasm and success:

> Patients notice when their nurses enjoy their work. When one staff member is busy, another one pitches in to help. Confident and autonomous nurses, who address patient needs immediately, ensure patient satisfaction. Many physicians prefer this kind of facility because they want their patients to experience quality care.
>
> Positive environments are responsible for success stories in many venues: Positive environments result in strong families. Parents and their children view their home as a relaxing sanctuary. They feel safe while exploring new challenges, secure in the knowledge that they will have support even with failure. Mutual trust enables all of the family members to live up to their full potential.

Notice the way that the following professional organization enables its members to reach new heights:

The organization has set high standards and keeps raising the bar to motivate its members to choose difficult goals. Veteran members generously support new people by sharing their expertise. This builds commitment and enables the members to return support to the organization that welcomed them so warmly when they were the new ones.

Words that describe positive cultures include supportive, generous, confident, sharing, warm, safe, secure, trusting, excellent, achieving, and collaborating.

CEOs drive health care cultures. Consider Frank, CEO of the fictional Expertise Hospital System. He sets the tone for the whole organization. He sincerely respects the work of every employee and exhibits a supportive attitude during staff interactions. He shares power and encourages other managers to follow his lead, to treat employees fairly. This means that the managers encourage staff at all levels to contribute their ideas. Managers feel proud of the way their direct-care staff have raised patient satisfaction and reduced medical errors. Frank has a congenial style and often takes the time for casual conversations with nurses and other staff. Employees have a strong sense of loyalty to him and to the whole organization. As a result, employees are consistently more productive than those at nearby facilities with a negative culture.

Researchers from Princeton, Stanford, and Berkley, studying productive companies around the world, found that companies with high productivity use similar strategies.

"In highly productive companies, the cultures studied were all based on the same set of standards" (Jennings, 2002), including the following:

- A set of deeply held values
- An environment where the work follows "best practices," as determined by those involved in completing the job
- A shared collective ambition to eliminate waste and achieve high productivity

Keeping Patients Safe: Transforming the Work Environment of Nurses, the November 2003 report by the Institute of Medicine (IOM) of the National Academies (2004), focused on the environment in which nurses work and on the culture that surrounds them:

"The health care workforce needs to be substantially transformed to better protect patients from health care errors," says a new report from the IOM of the National Academies. The report calls for changes in how nurse staffing levels are established and for mandatory limits on nurses' work hours, as part of a comprehensive plan to reduce problems that threaten patient safety by strengthening the work environment in four areas: management, workforce deployment, work design, and organizational culture.

"No one or two actions by themselves can keep patients safe," said Donald M. Steinwachs, chair of the committee that wrote the report. "Rather, creating work environments that reduce errors and increase patient safety will require fundamental changes in how nurses work, how they are deployed, and how the very culture of the organization understands and acts on safety." (IOM, 2004)

Consider this situation, in which staff collaborated to prevent errors:

A nurse discovers that a patient's address book has been lost. She is upset about the patient's loss and initiates a brainstorming session with the other team members. They come up with an idea that simplifies the management and labeling of patient belongings. After the change, the charge nurse leaves the following note for the nurse manager: "This was the problem, and this is how we solved it. FYI."

After applying the innovation, there were no lost belongings for more than two years, which represented a quality-enhancing and cost-effective result for an hour's worth of work by five people.

The problem was completely solved and needed no follow-up by the nurse manager. These empowered staff members saved significant management time. Empowered nurses enabled the manager to increase his own productivity. Organizational support of nurse autonomy resulted in high quality care, reduced risk, and effective teamwork.

Empowered nurses save management time.

The Magnet hospital program endorses positive cultures by strengthening the connection between positive cultures and patient-care excellence. Magnet facilities promote nurse autonomy by showcasing the results of patient and nurse satisfaction. Nursing leaders from Magnet hospitals express the importance of culture. As nurse leaders involved in various research studies reported,

> A supportive organization sends the message loud and clear that nurses are its most crucial asset and that providing excellence in patient care is the most crucial outcome. Good patient care comes from satisfied nurses, and you can't get that order mixed up. (Upenieks, 2003)

"Good patient care comes from satisfied nurses."
—Magnet hospital nurse leaders

Organizations that promote nurse satisfaction provide the best patient care; those with the opposite approach end up draining away employee energy. Read what Barbara Reinhold, PhD, says about negative cultures in her book *Toxic Work*: "Toxic work situations sap your energy . . . then the insidious eating away of energy and self-esteem begins in earnest" (Reinhold, 1996).

As frontline direct-care employees, nurses can work smarter by generating ideas that make their jobs easier without losing quality. Nurses working in negative cultures, keep those ideas to themselves. One way to improve nurse morale is to give nurses the power to improve their work environment.

Before the shortage, nurses who suggested improvements were ridiculed and considered to be expendable. As a result, nurses kept their silence. It was only after there were fewer nurses available to hire that organizations tried to reduce their nurse turnover. But by then, many nurses had already left the health care industry.

Consider how the following CEO's expectations have cost his facility a sizeable amount of money. When asked about nursing turnover, a long-term-care CEO replied, "Oh, we're doing great. We've lowered our nurse turnover rate from 70% to 30% a year."

My question was, "That's certainly a step in the right direction, but do you realize that every time you lose a nurse, you lose about $50,000?" As he multiplied $50,000 by the number of nurses that he had recently lost, he replied, "I never thought of it that way."

Relationship management is one of the best ways to improve organizational cultures. Review the following three guiding principles of management to see how they can assist you to build a committed and loyal staff:

1. Leaders and managers are more effective when they build strong relationships with their staff.

2. Organizations that provide environments in which nurses can perform at their best attract and retain the best people.
3. Long-term strategies, such as effective communication and staff-friendly cultures, enable organizations to achieve the best results.

Building positive relationships is one of the best no-cost strategies to improve health care. Building solid relationships and developing a sense of trust are so important. Think about your own life. Who are the people you trust? What attributes do they have that determine trustworthiness?

Write the numbers 1 to 10 on a piece of paper. List the 10 most important qualities that describe the people that you trust. Those are the qualities to develop within you. Your list may include dependability, sincerity, and a caring attitude. Ask other people about what is on their list. Then add those qualities to your own list and use the list as your guide to becoming more trustworthy. Add the element of time: people usually wait a while before trusting someone; they want to see how consistent you are.

People are more likely to trust when each side displays a consistent code of ethical behavior. Some people want to improve trust, but they don't want to make the first move. Trusting makes people vulnerable. If they have been burned in the past, they are reluctant to have it happen again. The first step in building trust is to scrap your obsolete power structure. All health care professionals are equally important, and everyone should be treated with respect. Listening is the second step. Listen with an open mind and without preconceived ideas that distort what you hear. Review the following list of specific descriptors for trusting relationships between managers and clinical staff.

- Managers and staff value their differences as assets to use for the patient's benefit.
- Staff and managers work as partners.
- They share the same vision.
- Managers empower their staff.
- Clinical staff and managers are both accountable for results.
- They enjoy mutual respect.
- They produce quality care.
- Managers address errors promptly so that each person involved can discover all of the relevant facts.
- Managers avoid using fear and punishment. They substitute relationships, communication, and education instead.

With trust and good communication, managers are able to start building commitment. Commitment enables you to build a culture in which people feel free to "be themselves" as they work together. This kind of freedom enables staff members to use their full professional capacity and to share their knowledge for the good of the whole organization.

An ambulatory care nurse notices the specific education needs of a patient in the emergency room. He addresses the patient's need with a customized and comprehensive patient education plan that will prevent future ER visits. This response would not have been possible in a negative culture. Fast-paced ER environments leave little time for patient education. Many ER nurses are unable to spend time and energy on education because most of their time and energy is consumed by a negative workplace and a long line of people in ER waiting rooms.

To function as a mature professional, ask yourself the following questions:

- When did I last say "Thank you" to a coworker?
- Do I listen when my peers try to communicate?
- How often do I ask my peers whether I can help them complete their assignment?

Working in a positive culture means using your sense of humor. Humor deepens relationships and relieves stress. Think back to a time when you shared a good laugh with a coworker. Didn't you feel more relaxed? Haven't you felt stronger relationships with people who make you laugh? The next time that you attend a corporate event, notice which departments are having the most fun. They are usually the ones receiving the most awards; humor promotes productivity and quality.

You can also use humor as a vehicle to deliver negative news. Humor is like a parachute—it gives negative information a soft landing. However, this only happens if you use humor skillfully and with sensitivity.

Humor is like a parachute. It gives negative information a soft landing.

Ten suggestions to promote a positive culture:

1. Invite new nurses to join you for breaks and meals.
2. Start a support group for new nurses.

3. Become a preceptor. If you are already a preceptor, take a refresher course to improve your skills.
4. Request the education department to bring new nurses together to express both positive and negative feelings.
5. Be a good role model for others.
6. Support effort as well as success.
7. Give encouragement when someone tackles a difficult assignment.
8. Collaborate to obtain feedback and improve care. Support other people's projects. Be as enthusiastic about their projects as you are about your own.
9. Increase your own self-respect. How can nurses ask for the respect of others if they don't respect themselves? Our self-image influences our treatment of others. When defensive, we perceive situations selectively and assume that the results will be negative.
10. Cultivate a win-win attitude. Exhibit an attitude of abundance. Encourage your peers to contribute their full potential. Embracing differences enable us to use everyone's ideas to resolve health care challenges.

Well-treated employees promote patient satisfaction. For example, managed-care organizations (MCOs) have an opportunity to support strong customer service. This means providing education for patients and supporting them through difficult times.

Health care organizations interact with many groups: patients, families, employees, providers, physicians, the government, and insurance companies. Keeping an open mind enables staff to represent their company as compassionate, knowledgeable, and progressive. A positive culture is an opportunity to project your best image.

Promoting a Staff-Friendly Culture

TIPS FOR CLINICAL NURSES

- Maintain a positive attitude.
- Contribute your ideas at work.
- Support your peers.
- Value your nursing contributions.
- Teach others to treat you with respect.

TIPS FOR MANAGERS

- Be knowledgeable about group dynamics.
- Support cooperation.
- Put nurse innovations into effect within 24 hours or as soon as possible.
- Create a positive environment.
- Recognize that nurses are high-value human resources.

TIPS FOR EDUCATORS

- Assess your students' potentials and seek to fulfill them.
- Provide an open learning environment.
- Be knowledgeable about collaboration.
- Show students how culture affects nursing care.
- Collaborate with clinical nurses and managers.

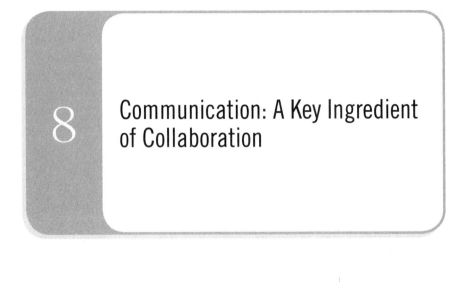

Communication: A Key Ingredient of Collaboration

Communication works for those who work at it. —*John Powell*

CONVERSATIONS

One of my most important conversations was one that I had with myself when I gave up my comfort zones. I decided to become skilled at public speaking and writing for publication after I realized that the pain of remaining silent was greater than the discomfort of conquering my fears. Communication leverages our clinical skills and it feels good to work for patient safety and nurse staffing in a larger arena.

This chapter includes new skills as well as different approaches to skills that you may already have: assertiveness, small talk, public speaking, writing, effective clinical communication, body language, customizing communication messages, and negotiation.

Add your own personality and style to these skills and make them your own. And, consider having that conversation with yourself about leaving those comfort zones behind. Listen to what Gerry Spence, an attorney who never lost a criminal trial, says about fear: "Fear is energy that is convertible to power—our power" (Spence, 1995). Honing your communication skills gives you power.

Factors That Affect Communication

Communication involves many variables. It's not just what you say, it's how you say it, and, most of all, it's your credibility that determines whether people pay attention. One way to change communication dynamics is to change the venue, the location, of the talks; environments make a big difference. For instance, an informal retreat environment probably stimulates creativity better than an everyday office.

Power differentials and time constraints also affect communication. Having a level playing field where employees at every level have the same amount of power facilitates understanding. Sometimes a deadline is helpful, but tight time constraints can interfere with quality when people feel too rushed.

A 2004 study of 3,500 randomly selected RNs revealed that a clear majority perceived that the nursing shortage had resulted in increased communication problems (Beurhaus, Donelin, Ulrich, Norman, & Dittus, 2005).

One problem with communication that relates to staffing issues occurs when both sides become very polarized and distrustful. Even a small amount of insincerity on either side negates substantial tangible offerings, such as premium pay and bonuses.

HOW IS COMMUNICATION LIKE ROMANCE?

Perhaps one way to view the complexities of communication is by comparing communication to romance—another common life experience that could also be considered an art.

How would you answer the following 10 questions? (Note that I have answered some of the following questions for myself. Your answers may be different.)

1. Are there any hard and fast rules for romance? No
2. Does romance depend mostly on relationships? Yes
3. Is every romance different? Yes
4. Does the fact that you sent flowers or candy necessarily ensure a successful romance? No
5. Can a small amount of insincerity undo a large quantity of tangible offerings (candy and flowers)? Yes
6. Should even small amounts of abusive behavior be enough to end the relationship? Yes

7. Is consistency important? Yes
8. Can you improve your romantic skills by learning from your failures as well as your successes? Yes
9. Is romance an art? Yes
10. Is romance worth the effort? You have to decide that one for yourself.

If your employees view you as insincere, it really doesn't matter what else you do. Insincerity leads to a lack of credibility, resulting in your communication efforts being ignored. In other words, sincerity and credibility are necessary foundations for communication effort. Without a strong foundation of credibility, your communication efforts will crumble even if you say the right words.

Most health care professionals could improve their communication skills. During their coffee breaks, nurses complain to each other, but not often enough to those with the power to make changes.

The nursing crisis has given nurses center stage. Rising to this challenge requires activation of creativity and communication to make our case. The rewards are great: respect, influence, and professional fulfillment.

Communication Skills for Nurses

Although nurses are skilled with informal nurse-patient communication, many nurses need to expand their communication repertoire with the following skills.

Assertiveness

Assertiveness is an important part of effective communication. In the past, managers disciplined assertive nurses, but the nursing shortage has given nurses leverage. Now is the right time for nurses to ask for what they need. Discarding negativity is not easy, but negativity stimulates a response of more negativity. Disarming the other side is more practical. You can disarm individuals on the other side by carefully listening to their thoughts and asking relevant, nonthreatening questions to help you understand the specifics of what they want. Once you have disarmed the other side, you can make your own case and state your needs. Here are some suggestions:

- Intervene calmly and confidently.
- Respond to problems in a timely way, to avoid overreaction to small incidents.

- Clearly articulate the importance of nursing perspectives.
- Use language that management understands.

"I" statements are important when communicating your thoughts and feelings. But when persuading others to accept your viewpoint, "you" statements often work better because they describe benefits that may interest the other side. For example, you could say, "I don't like this policy, and I don't think that many other nurses will like it either." But it would be better to say, "Using this policy will result in the loss of at least three nurses, costing you over $150,000." Or "This change will increase medical errors, drive patients away, and lower your accreditation score." You will be more likely to be successful with the "you" format.

A structured way to understand each side's viewpoint is to use the following worksheet. You can use this worksheet with any issue when you might have trouble understanding the other side.

Worksheet 8.1

Clinical nurses needs:	Issue	Management needs
Enough time to be able to provide safe care for patients	Patient safety	Maintain accreditation and a good reputation to serve the community
Enough nurses to ensure quality care	Nurse staffing	Attract and retain nurses with good critical thinking skills.

Statement of my perspective:

_____

_____

_____

Statement of the perspective of the other side:

_____

_____

_____

Small Talk

Small talk is an important strength. Small talk builds rapport and makes your messages more compelling. Shy people, who have difficulty engaging in small talk, can improve if they are willing to learn new skills, such as the following:

- Read books on small talk, such as *What Do I Say Next?* by Susan Roane (1997).
- Prepare for small talk by reading magazines and newspapers and choosing a few topics to talk about.
- Prepare a few questions that are likely to get other people to talk. For instance, ask open-ended questions about common topics, such as favorite vacations, books, and hobbies. Answers to these questions give you clues about the other person's interests, enabling you to follow up with more specific questions to continue the conversation.

Public Speaking

Solid public-speaking skills make you more visible, an antidote to nurse powerlessness. With public speaking, you can influence many people at the same time. Consider the following example of an employee who enjoyed a rapid rise to high management:

Amy was a supervisor who recognized the value of public speaking. She joined Toastmasters (www.toastmasters.org), where she had the opportunity to practice her public-speaking skills. She also gained experience as the master of ceremonies for meetings.

Amy used her public speaking skills to develop an effective training program for her employees. Her manager recognized her initiative and praised the way she had inspired employee excellence. Amy's manager had planned to emcee a retirement party for a high-level manager, but she was called away at the last minute by a serious family illness. She asked Amy to take her place because she knew that Amy was an experienced public speaker.

Amy had an opportunity to showcase her speaking skills in front of many senior managers. Shortly after Amy's successful stint as an emcee, she was asked to rotate to several key corporate positions. After her positive performance in these positions, Amy received a promotion to an important high-level management job.

Writing for Publication

Writing is another learnable skill that provides the opportunity to influence many people with one effort. Joining a writers group (most areas have local writers groups) is a good way to learn to write like a journalist. Why is writing like a journalist important? Learning to write like a journalist is the best way for nurses to ensure that their ideas are communicated in the most effective way. It takes practice, but you will find that there are many opportunities for nurses who are good writers.

What happens when you attend a writers group? Attendees bring a copy of their written piece for each member of the group, and the members critique each others' work. Rewriting your piece based on this critique enables you to improve your writing. Writers groups are also good places to learn about the publication process.

Whether you are speaking in public or writing an article, using numbers dramatizes your issue. For instance, saying "Reducing nurse turnover by a mere 3% saves a 300-bed hospital over $500,000 annually" is more effective than saying, "You save money if you lower nurse turnover."

Apply Your Communication Skills

1. Break the code of silence. Nurses have experienced an informal code of silence when prior communication attempts resulted in reprisals. Many nurses have learned that it is safer to keep their opinions to themselves; nursing input is lost as a result.
2. Earn the trust of others. Reliability and consistency are what others look for.
3. Listen. Another way to improve communication is to listen. Some of the advantages of listening are the following:
   - Identifying problems.
   - Exposing feelings—those invaluable but sometimes inconvenient traits that make us truly human. We need to manage our feelings and give them a positive focus instead of having to deny them.
   - Jump-starting the solution process; answers pop up during candid conversations.

- Relieving stress. Bottling up thoughts and feelings only depletes energy.
- Disarming the other person and making it easier to achieve your goals (as mentioned earlier in this chapter).

Clinical Communication Models

SBAR Communication Model

This model was developed by Kaiser Permanente to facilitate communication between health care professionals. It is especially useful when staff are reporting changes in a patient's condition, and it was also intended to be a communication model for teams. It is now in common use in many health care facilities across the country.

The SBAR acronym stands for the following:

Situation: The situation is an "in the moment" description of the situation (e.g., Mr. Smith developed chest pain 10 minutes ago).

Background: Relevant information that led up to the situation (e.g., Mr. Smith had been visiting with his family).

Assessment: Subjective and objective measure of the patient and the situation (e.g., Mr. Smith does not have a history of gastro-esophageal reflux disease [GERD]).

Recommendation: What you think should be done (e.g., perhaps an electrocardiogram).

Advantages: Having a model that is familiar to both professionals is helpful. The model provides an opportunity to transfer a sizeable amount of relevant information within a short period of time. It lends itself to respect for nurses because it provides an opportunity for nurses to give their assessments and recommendations.

Disadvantages: As with other good tools, SBAR can be misused. In situations with strong power differentials, the model can be a source of conflict. For instance, each professional can have a different expectation of how extensive the situation or background descriptions should be. Each participant may also have a different idea of what information he or she considers to be relevant, resulting in criticism instead of the asking of respectful questions. Excessive stress, such as

BEST PRACTICE: THE GREAT LISTENING MODEL

Beth Boynton, RN, MS, Nurse Trainer, Coach, Consultant, Speaker, York Beach, ME

The Great Listening model was designed to help facilities comply with the requirement of the Joint Commission (TJC) for structured communication during "hand-offs" and to enhance the Joint Commission "speak-up" campaign, which encourages self-advocacy and assertiveness for patients. It can be used and modified according to organizational needs and preferences. Effective listening is sometimes simple and sometimes complex—but always essential.

Greeting: Hi, (person's name). This is a simple, quick, and respectful way to begin a stressful conversation.

Respectful listening: When communicating with someone with lesser power, realize that the other person may have anxiety about bringing a concern up the ladder; yet, this is exactly what clinicians are supposed to do.

Review: A quick summary of the information can clarify the reporter's concerns and allow for additional thoughts. A few seconds at this point can lead to clinicians feeling heard, respected, and, ultimately, understood.

Recommend or request more information: At this stage, the responder has enough information to initiate an order or to gather more information.

Reward: Statements such as "Thank you for your attention to this patient's needs," "I appreciate your call," or "Call me if problems persist" demonstrate respect for the reporter and contribute to an atmosphere of teamwork.

during a life-threatening emergency, can be one of the root causes of SBAR misuse.

Use Body Language Effectively

Nonverbal communication accounts for more than half of your message, with some estimates topping 90%. Observe body language to detect what others might be feeling. Nurses who work in negative environments absorb much of that negativity. Because any human being can tolerate only so much negativity, many nurses struggle not to pass that negativity on to patients. This is why managers should treat nurses the same way that they would like their nurses to treat the patients. Nurses are internal customers; patients are external customers. Both types of customers are important.

Use Different Communication Approaches for Different People

Ask yourself the following questions: Does the staff represent a variety of personality styles and cultural backgrounds? Do I use the same approach for everyone? Is my approach based on my own needs? If you answered yes to any of these questions, consider using multiple approaches for different people. If you know, for example, that a staff member is gregarious and extroverted, use a gregarious approach. On the other hand, a staff member with quiet self-confidence may respond best to a calm, logical, and systematic approach. Managers and nurses with a variety of communication styles can improve their relationships and are more likely to achieve exceptional patient outcomes.

ACTIVITIES TO IMPROVE YOUR COMMUNICATION SKILLS

1. Assess your image and make a list of self-description adjectives. Ask others to make a similar list about you. How do the lists compare?
2. Keep a journal for 30 days about your overall communication results. Try to spot if you have a communication pattern. You can also include comments from other managers and staff when analyzing your pattern.
3. Keep a communication log of your informal conversations with nurses for the next 30 days. Record the tone of those conversations. Were they warm and genial? Did you talk with nurses on all shifts? Who initiated each conversation? Then decide whether you used informal conversations effectively. Informal conversations serve multiple purposes:
   - Assessing attitudes
   - Developing rapport
   - Giving attention
   - Discovering needs
   - Understanding goals
   - Validating feelings
   - Providing support
   - Giving praise
   - Correcting actions
   - Finding facts
   - Expressing self-disclosure

If you have too few informal conversations, improve your availability by scheduling unstructured time with staff.

Nurses Are the Best Marketers

During conversations with nurses, acknowledge their value beyond clinical functions. Consider using nurses as marketers:

- Start a conversation in a staff meeting about nursing's role in your facility.
- Dedicate a portion of your staff meetings to listing current challenges. Then brainstorm about the opportunities that lie beyond the challenges.

An example of an opportunity lying beyond a challenge is the following example, which describes a missed marketing opportunity by hospitals. The first subacute units, which appeared in the 1990s, cared for a patient population consisting of people who had no place to go— patients who were not appropriate for home care, long-term care, or acute hospitalization. Independent subacute companies provided a less expensive alternative for complex but stable patients with medical or surgical, rehabilitation, or oncology needs. Hospitals themselves eventually created subacute or transitional units. However, they could have been first in this market if there had been better communication between CEOs and nurses. Nurses and social workers had experienced frustration for a long time when trying to find facilities for these patients. With better communication, hospitals would have recognized this situation as a marketing opportunity and could have been the first to open subacute units.

People don't always realize that communication lessons occur around them every day. Learn to pay attention to the way that people communicate in meetings, at home, in grocery stores. Listen to your favorite teenager. The sources are endless.

A group leader wanted to encourage one of her members to volunteer to bring refreshments to the next meeting. When no volunteers were forthcoming, she asked them the following question: "If you were going to bring refreshments, what would you bring?" She then asked the group to take a vote on their favorite refreshment choice. We all had a good laugh, and of course, someone volunteered to bring refreshments.

I quickly added the leader's "If you were . . ." question to my communication tool kit.

Miscommunication is often harmful, but it can be humorous as well. Because I sometimes include a book raffle in my education programs, I called a bookstore and asked the clerk if they carried *The Wisdom of Teams*. She answered by saying, "Well, that's an oxymoron if I've ever heard one." I quickly realized that she must have thought that I had asked for "The Wisdom of *Teens*"; she must have had a bad time with her teenager that day. We both had a good laugh and commiserated about the challenges of raising adolescents. There was more than a grain of truth in this situation. Many teens can be very wise and can be good communication role models for adults. Many teens are authentic, empathetic, compassionate, and caring; many adults have replaced these essential qualities with cynicism.

Negotiation

People negotiate every single day; parents negotiate with their children, merchants negotiate with their customers, and nations negotiate with each other. Knowing how to be a good negotiator is an important skill for nurses. Solid negotiating has often eluded nurses because powerlessness has made stating an opinion quite risky. As the working conditions of nurses deteriorated, nurses negotiated by using their only bargaining chip: they voted with their feet and walked out of health care.

As diversity increases, staff members need to improve their negotiation skills if they expect to bring people together instead of driving them apart. Conflict is inevitable whenever a variety of people work together, yet many fail to realize that conflict can be a positive force. Conflict is positive when you respect all opinions and combine many perspectives in innovative ways. Consider what Sy Landau states in his book *From Conflict to Creativity: How Resolving Workplace Disagreements Can Inspire Innovation and Productivity*: "Without the catalyst of fresh ideas and differing perspectives, change and growth are not possible" (Landau, 2001).

Successful negotiators are skillful relationship builders. They nurture trust and build bridges. Strengthening the negotiating skills of clinical staff strengthens the whole organization because negotiation is one of the ways to bring clinical issues to the boardroom.

Many negotiation experts advocate the following principles:

1. Research what is important to the other side before you start your negotiations.
2. Ask questions to discover new information to add to your initial research and impression.
3. Build relationships. One way to do this is to talk about what you both already agree about.
4. Use empathy to disarm the other side. I have a favorite statement that I call "the magic sentence." This magic sentence can solve multiple problems: get your car fixed properly, teach responsibility to your children, or succeed in almost any other circumstances. It starts with an empathetic phrase. An example of using this sentence is, "I know that _____ is difficult (or frustrating), but it is your responsibility to _____" (Burns, 1980).
   Some examples of ways to use this sentence:
   - Parent to child: "I know that algebra is difficult, but it is your responsibility to take the time to do your best."
   - Clinical nurse to manager: "I know that staffing is difficult, but it is your responsibility to provide enough staff to maintain patient safety."
   - Manager to clinical staff: "I know that being away from family is difficult, but it is your responsibility to work your share of the holidays."
5. Find a common purpose. During one difficult negotiation, representatives from each side were asked to spend 60 minutes in separate rooms to write their common purpose on a flip chart. When they were done and compared the two charts, the lists were practically identical.
6. Think long term: a long-term approach adds time for relationship building.
7. Have a plan. You may not be able to have everything your way, but planning enables you to prioritize what is important to you.
8. Avoid inflammatory words. Why destroy your chances for success with careless comments?
9. Think win-win: coming to an agreement that works for both sides enables you to continue working together over the long term.
10. Avoid assumptions. Noticing body language is important, but it is only a start. Validate your impression with questions.

11. Pick your battles. Focus on what is most important. Some issues are too minor to bother with. If you divide your energy into minute pieces, you may not be able to achieve your most important goals.

12. Use the "flinch." When someone from the other side makes a statement, act shocked (exaggerate how shocked you are) and remain silent. Many times, the other person will back off.

13. Let someone from the other side speak first. A common motto is, "He who speaks first, loses."

14. Use diffusion. I first experienced diffusion when my firstborn child started nursery school. One teacher, very experienced and loving with her small charges, had a favorite phrase that she always used when she denied a child's request. She would just say, "Tomorrow is another day." Because the children couldn't argue with that statement, they would accept it as an answer and calmly walk away without feeling defeated. That's diffusion— making a statement with which everyone has to agree. Using diffusion and making a statement such as "The patients need a variety of caregivers" might bring a diverse health care team together.

15. Increase the size of the "pie." If your budget is too small, generate more revenue (bake more pies) instead of always decreasing expenses (cutting smaller and smaller pieces of pie). Consider the following example: Many nursing organizations have lost members, reducing their dues income, an important source of revenue. As responsible professionals, they want to balance the budget. But if cutting member benefits interferes with recruitment and retention, offering more benefits may work better because benefits increase the value of membership.

    Consider how the following free or inexpensive benefits can be valuable to others. You may be able to strike an agreement by offering one of these benefits in almost any negotiation.

    ■ Networking opportunities
    ■ Mentors
    ■ Leadership experience
    ■ Professional support
    ■ Collective action on common problems
    ■ Support for innovation
    ■ Group purchasing

Promoting Effective Communication

TIPS FOR CLINICAL NURSES

- Eliminate the code of silence.
- Learn to speak and write for publication.
- Be assertive in appropriate situations.
- Have positive expectations.
- Build your small-talk skills.

TIPS FOR MANAGERS

- Earn your staff's credibility.
- Encourage nurses to network with each other.
- Respond to communication problems promptly.
- Encourage staff participation.
- Raise productivity with good communication.

TIPS FOR EDUCATORS

- Include communication as a major part of your curriculum.
- Teach negotiation skills.
- Support the value of speaking in public and writing for publication.
- Show students the importance of nonverbal communication.
- Use experiential learning experiences.

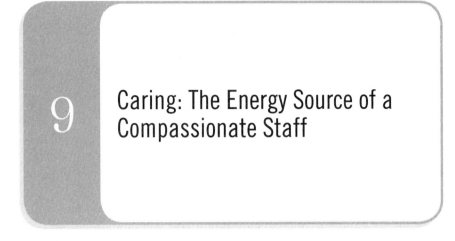

9 Caring: The Energy Source of a Compassionate Staff

The caring energy produced in caring organizational contexts, drives productivity. *—Riane Eisler*

People exchange psychic energy when they form and maintain relationships. I rediscovered this process for myself, after becoming a professional speaker, by noticing the presence of mutual energy exchanges with audiences. The same exchange occurs in nurse-patient, family, and other loving interactions. Nurse-patient relationships refresh both staff and patients when energy flows back and forth.

The loss of nurse-patient relationships triggers burnout and low nurse productivity. If nurses must rush through patient care, energy only flows from the nurse; none flows back, resulting in a serious energy deficit that eventually causes burnout.

Consider how the following research delineates the limits of the human capacity for empathy.

How good are Good Samaritans in a hurry? A team of social psychologists staged a powerful demonstration that the failure to help strangers in distress is due more to situational variables than to personal values. A number of theology students were directed to tape a sermon about the Good Samaritan at a taping center. On the way to the taping center was a stranger (an actor) huddled up in an alley on the ground, moaning in dire distress.

Students were randomly told either that they should hurry because they were late or that they had enough time. The result was that 90% of the students, who were told to rush, passed up the chance to be a Good Samaritan because they were in a hurry to give a sermon on it. The more time the seminarians thought that they had, the more likely they were to stop and help. This research was replicated when the same result occurred a second time. (Zimbardo, 2007)

The only variable in this experiment was the time-pressured environment, because seminarians were already viewed as being empathetic. So we can extrapolate that our time-pressured health care environment may also interfere with nurse empathy.

Neuroscientist Debra Niehoff has documented that the neurochemistry of stress makes it harder to be conscious of others or even fully conscious of oneself: "Empathy takes a back seat to relief from the numbing discomfort of a stress-deadened nervous system" (Eisler, 2007).

The evidence suggests that we need to make it possible for our nurses to have the time to care, to be able to use their natural empathy as they care for patients, so that they don't experience the "numbing discomfort" of the stress-deadened nervous system described by Niehoff. Nurses are the caregivers of our nation's most vulnerable people; patients need the empathy of our caring nurses.

An important benefit of practicing within a caring profession is the effect on the caregivers themselves. True loving relationships are thought to expand ego boundaries, permanently increasing one's future capacity to love (Peck, 1978) . It's the same for caring. As a result of caring connections, many nurses experience significant growth in their total capacity to care, but this process is blocked when burnout results in emotional exhaustion.

Caring Raises Nurse Productivity

- Nurses experience a surge of self-respect when they are proud of their accomplishments. This surge results in increased nurse productivity.
- Nurses with enough time to care radiate a sense of calm, thereby reducing patient and staff anxiety. One of the most difficult parts of coping with a serious illness is the uncertainty. Caring nurses

transmit calming energy, to help patients relieve stress and, at the same time, to support high staff productivity.

- Having time to care improves the physical health of nurses, enabling them to be energized and raising productivity.
- With enough time, nurses are able to work smarter by planning their work, rather than having to spend most of their time managing crises.

Working in a caring environment improves a nurse's ability to problem-solve, as described by Riane Eisler in *The Real Wealth of Nations*, recognizing empathy as a major component of caring and recognizing that stress "inhibits our capacity for perceiving alternatives . . . As stress expert Bruce McEwen puts it, 'people say that stress makes you stupid. But what it really does is limit your options'" (Eisler, 2007).

Books such as *Power vs. Force* by David R. Hawkins, MD, PhD, describe how energy fields bathe others with positive energy from emotions such as hope. Low energy fields, based on emotions such as fear, also spread to others. That is why caring nurses have such calming effects on others.

Caring nurses also have more patience, and patience becomes even more important as our patient population continues to age. Walking an 80-year-old patient to the bathroom can be time-consuming; in the future, nurses will need more time, not less, to care for their patients.

How Can Organizations Increase Their Support of Caring Staff

The Influence of Caring Science

A number of nurse leaders have come forward with the results of their deep inquiry into caring. One of these leaders is Jean Watson. Watson's Theory of Human Caring has continued to evolve since its inception in the late 1970s. Transpersonal caring relationships move beyond the ego-self—radiating spiritual, even cosmic connections that tap into a patient's healing potential. Transpersonal caring seeks to connect with and embrace the spirit or soul of the other in the authentic relationship moment (Watson, 2005).

Here are some of Watson's tenets of transpersonal care:

- Transpersonal caring is communicated via the practitioner's authentic presence in a caring relationship.
- A transpersonal caring relationship connotes a spirit-to-spirit unitary connection within a caring moment.
- Transpersonal caring promotes self-knowledge, self-control, and self-healing patterns and possibilities (Watson, 2005).

Mihaly Czikszentmihalyi, a psychologist and expert on "flow," describes going beyond the ego:

> While one typically forgets the self during the flow experience, after the event, a person's self-esteem reappears in a stronger form than it had been before . . . Similarly, people who have more flow experiences also have higher self-esteem overall. While unexpected, this paradoxical finding is not really surprising. Half a century ago, the Austrian psychiatrist Viktor Frankl wrote that happiness cannot be attained by wanting to be happy—it must come as the unintended consequence of working for a goal greater than oneself. (Czikszentmihalyi, 2005)

Mother Teresa's mission to bring comfort to the poor and dying population in India was greater than herself. Each of her small acts of caring was part of a greater legacy of love that she left for the world.

Patients need caring environments because physical ailments heal more quickly when patients' minds and bodies are able to connect. Caring provides a milieu in which healing energy combines with physical medicine, thereby improving patient outcomes. Caring is mutually beneficial, for both patient and caregiver, and preserves the holistic health of both.

Poet and author David Whyte views work as a pilgrimage of our identity. He expresses concern about losing our identity. "Our bodies can be present in our work, but our hearts, minds and imaginations can be placed firmly in neutral or engaged elsewhere" (Whyte, 2001).

Just as for patients, a caring environment enables nurses to be physically, emotionally, and spiritually well. Healthy staff members are more resilient than those who are chronically fatigued; healthy nurses are able to reach peak activity levels without difficulty.

Promoting Caring

TIPS FOR CLINICAL NURSES

- Support other caring nurses.
- Care for yourself.
- Keep up with caring science.
- Expand your relationships.
- Speak up for caring.

TIPS FOR MANAGERS

- Provide staff with time to care.
- Praise caring acts.
- Understand that staff energy depends on caring.
- Speak up to senior managers and trustees about caring.
- Be a caring manager.

TIPS FOR EDUCATORS

- Teach the importance of caring.
- Engage students in research on caring.
- Be a caring educator.
- Educate students regarding the physiological response to caring.
- Bring caring science experiences to others.

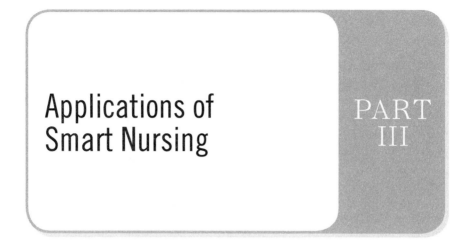

Applications of Smart Nursing

PART III

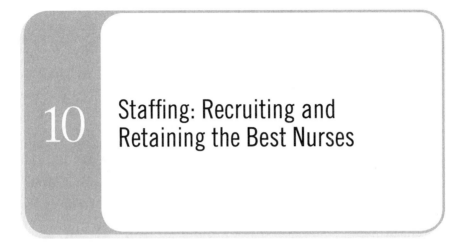

10   Staffing: Recruiting and Retaining the Best Nurses

We need to learn how to engage the creativity that exists everywhere in our organizations.   —*Margaret J. Wheatley*

STAFFING CHALLENGES

Health care managers are spending an inordinate amount of time on staffing. Constant staff changes prevent them from moving forward (see Figure 10.1), leaving little time for proactive actions such as strategic planning and progressive staff development. As a result, they must close units or delay launching new services.

Recent estimates of RN turnover (per nurse) range from $63,100 to 67,100 (Jones, 2004) the costs of nurse turnover, Part 2). Studies also link high staff turnover to reduced patient satisfaction (Jones, 2004).

Organizations often try to attract new patients with expensive advertising campaigns, but a positive workplace that attracts and retains competent staff is a better approach.

Those that try to manage nurses with coercion usually find that it makes matters worse. In his book *Primal Leadership*, Daniel Goleman gives a detailed description of the effects of coercion:

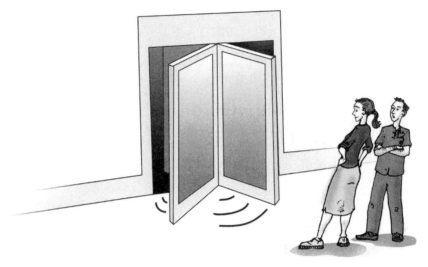

FIGURE 10.1 "Is this the door to the ER?"
"No, it's the door to HR. The nurses go in and out so fast you can't even see them."

The business world is rife with coercive leaders whose negative impact on those they lead has yet to catch up with them [. . .] When a major hospital system was losing money, the board hired a new president to turn the business around—and the effect was disastrous. As one physician told us, "He cut back staff mercilessly, especially in nursing. The hospital looked more profitable, but it was dangerously understaffed. . . . Everyone felt demoralized."

No surprise, then, that patient satisfaction ratings plummeted. When the hospital began to lose market share to its competition, the president grudgingly rehired many of the people he'd fired. "But to this day he's never admitted he was much too ruthless . . ." and he continues to manage by threat and intimidation. The nurses are back, but morale is not. Meanwhile, the president complains about patient satisfaction numbers—but fails to see that he's part of the problem (Goleman, 2002).

Nurses understand risk because they manage high-risk situations every day. Listening to nurses reduces overall risk because frontline employees notice safety problems early, in time to prevent catastrophic events.

It is not always necessary to increase staffing. Many times, rearranging staff provides better coverage. But moving nurses around causes problems. Nurses oppose floating because most nurses have encountered negative experiences, such as being floated without adequate preparation. Rather than risk their nursing license, nurses have simply refused to float.

Part of the solution is the intelligent use of cross-training. If you want cross-trained nurses, you will need to invest time, energy, and money. Schedule your nurses to work alongside experienced nurses in the new specialty. This involves duplicate staffing, resulting in higher short-term costs, but in the long-term, you will have greater staffing flexibility. You will need to give cross-trained nurses your support—tangible incentives such as higher salaries or vacation time, or intangible rewards such as higher status, desirable projects, or public recognition.

Magnet Force number 3 recommends using a participatory management style for staffing success. This Magnet force advises that nurses serving in leadership positions be visible and accessible to their staff. This principle also recommends that nursing leaders demonstrate how they value nursing feedback from all levels of their organization (ANCC). Magnet Force 4 recommends competitive salaries and flexible staffing models that support a safe and healthy work environment, which can be created with the involvement of direct-care nurses (ANCC). Magnet Force 5 recommends using professional models that promote nurse autonomy and accountability, focus on a patient's unique needs, and ensure that skilled nurses and adequate resources are available to accomplish the desired outcomes (ANCC).

Mandatory Overtime

Instead of arranging appropriate staffing, some organizations abuse mandatory overtime because it is convenient. An example is that of a nurse from the 11–7 shift who discovers that she has been mandated to work on the 7–3 shift. The nurse loses her right to have proper rest and her ability to ensure patient safety; fatigue causes medical errors and interferes with even a minimal life balance.

Most health care organizations spend more than $5 million per year on human resources. Some small organizations invest more than 75% of their budget on human resources. If you had a personal investment of $5 million in real estate or securities, you would no doubt spend time and energy to increase your return. Why not spend similar time and energy reducing the costs of human resources?

The nursing shortage has forced facilities to increase their staffing budgets to provide for "premium pay." Earning premium pay may sound profitable, but only in the short term. Nurses cannot sustain excessive mandatory overtime because it is physically and mentally exhausting.

Mandated shifts can also keep them from fulfilling their child care responsibilities. Consider the following two examples:

> At 2:00, a 7–3 shift nurse is told that she has to stay until 11:00. She is a single parent and must pick up her child from daycare at 5:00. This nurse is concerned because she takes her child care responsibilities seriously. Isn't she exactly the kind of nurse that we must keep in health care? Shouldn't we seek out and support nurses who take their responsibilities seriously? Aren't such nurses also the ones who will take their patient safety responsibilities seriously? When our coercive attitude toward mandatory overtime forces nurses to choose between being responsible parents and remaining in their profession, isn't something very wrong with a system that requests such a choice? Could this coercive attitude also be contributing to our escalating rate of medical errors?
>
> Another nurse working from 3 to 11 is told she must stay until 7:00 the next morning. She has two preschool children, and her husband works during the day, so she must now go all day without sleep until her husband comes home from work at 5:00. After working for 16 hours at a very demanding job, she must go without the rest that she needs.

Both of these nurses are likely to have high rates of illness and absenteeism and will eventually burn out. The short-term gain produced by premium pay quickly evaporates, and many of these nurses will ultimately leave health care for another occupation, thus deepening the nursing crisis.

Reversing Negative Situations

The nursing shortage is only a symptom. The real issue is that nurses are unable to improve their situation.

Health care organizations tend to react to crises, instead of acting before problems get out of hand. Some spend large amounts of money to recruit and train new nurses but spend little to retain them. More money doesn't help if nurses feel ashamed of the care that they give and, if no matter how hard they work, their professional effort isn't enough.

Senior managers, some with little or no clinical experience, create policies that nurses cannot follow in good conscience because they contradict sound nursing practice.

Inadequate Staffing

What happens when an organization cuts staffing without considering the consequences? Nurses, RNs and LPNs alike, then have responsibility without a voice. They have too little time to maintain even minimal safety standards. Nurses become concerned that they will miss important symptoms when there is little time for adequate observation or follow-up.

"Business as Usual" Versus Staff-Friendly Cultures

Long-Term Care in the "Business as Usual" Culture

Nonclinical people look at patient statistics in isolation, but nurses must look at the faces behind those numbers every day. For example, one of those faces belongs to Sarah, a resident of a long-term-care facility. She is frail, a shadow of the vibrant woman that she once was. You are a long-term care nurse. You would like to match the caring attitude of Sarah's family. You think about how much she is like your grandmother, whom you would want cared for with safety, dignity, and love. As you look Sarah in the eyes every day, you know that there is too little time to give her proper care.

You start to give morning medications to your 35 residents. You expect to finish your medication pass in about 2 hours, which gives you less than 3.5 minutes per person, not counting interruptions. In that 3.5 minutes, you must wash your hands, identify the patient, position the patient, correctly choose an average of 10 medications, crush those medications, and mix them with applesauce. As you administer those medications, you notice that Sarah only takes about a quarter of a teaspoon at a time. She also has 4 ounces of a nutritional supplement to drink. She only drinks a small sip at a time—about half a teaspoon—and then rests a second or two. You can do the math; it would take 10 to 15 minutes to administer just the supplement.

Facilities are penalized on accreditation reviews if their residents lose weight. Ordering supplements without providing enough time for the staff to administer them is an example of how facilities achieve high health-care compliance on paper records, coupled with low quality of care in actual practice.

So you do what you can in 3.5 minutes and then go on to the next resident. Physical assessments, assisting the LNA/CNAs, talking with staff and families, and telephoning physicians all take more time away from resident care.

Some facilities use agency or per diem nurses for every shift. Agency and per diem nurses are excellent, but they should fill specific staffing holes—not constitute most of the staff. Consider the result when a facility is entirely staffed with agency nurses. A 3-to-11 agency nurse in a long-term-care facility receives report from an agency nurse at 3 p.m. and gives report to another agency nurse at 11 p.m. All of the necessary tasks are carried out, but the residents don't even have the comfort of a familiar face. Such situations are as unfair to the agency nurses as they are to the residents. No matter how skilled the nurse, she or he needs to know something about each resident. How can an agency nurse identify changes in a resident's condition if no one in the facility has any idea about the resident's usual level of functioning? Agency nurses also become disenfranchised when they are unable to deliver high-quality care.

I received the following e-mail from a long-term-care nurse: "I, too, am experiencing the ravages of too little staff (1–2 LNAs, 1 nurse for 39 residents) and administration's indifference to our plight. After working for only six years as a nurse, I am on the edge of deciding to leave nursing."

Long-Term Care in a Staff-Friendly Culture

A better scenario for long-term care would be what Wilma receives. Wilma is a long-term resident whose son lives locally. However, her two daughters live out of state. Because both daughters are nurses, they manage the medical questions that arise. Staff turnover at Wilma's facility is very low, and the staff function as surrogate family members. When the LNA/CNAs pass Wilma's wheelchair, they stop and smile at her, pat her arm, and warmly say, "Wilma, you're looking good today. How are you?" Wilma smiles back. The LPN charge nurse, Sandra, knows both Wilma and her daughters well because she is a long-term employee. She anticipates the kind of information that the family members need to know and calls them periodically. Wilma's daughters are very appreciative that Sandy provides such personalized care and keeps them informed about their mother.

This is long-term care at its best. Low turnover and fair treatment of staff produce quality care, as well as financial viability for the facility. Families want their loved ones to be cared for in facilities such as this, which rarely have vacant beds.

A 2002 American Nurses Association (ANA) study found that 75% of nurses surveyed said the quality of care had declined in the past two years, and more than 4 out of 10 would not want their families to be patients at their facility because of the low-quality care (ANA, 2004).

Critical Care in the "Business as Usual" Culture

An Intensive Care Unit (ICU) nurse describes reporting for work and discovering that, instead of his usual one or two patients, he had been assigned four patients. His objections eventually were reflected by a negative comment on his evaluation.

Critical Care in a Staff-Friendly Culture

Ryan, an ICU nurse, has a two-patient assignment. Because the vents and A-lines require constant monitoring, he is very busy, but he is able to fulfill his assignment with safety and quality. He makes time, for example, to talk with the families of his patients and answer their questions. These families appreciate Ryan's support and his caring attitude. This makes their ordeal of living through a family member's life-threatening illness more bearable.

Home Care in the "Business as Usual" Culture

A home-care nurse finds that the increased workload prevents him from taking any morning or afternoon rest breaks. Lunch consists of driving through a fast-food restaurant and eating on the way back to work. Finally, after working since 8 a.m., he finds himself filling and programming a narcotic pain-control pump at 7:00 in the evening. Such pumps require exact attention and accuracy because they frequently run for 24 to 60 hours without further nursing examination. In such situations, any small error multiplies with time and can potentially result in a serious injury. The job requires the attention of an alert nurse.

Home Care in a Staff-Friendly Culture

Susan, a home-care nurse, has a full morning schedule of patient visits. Early on, she discovers medical complications that delay her, because she needed to call the physician. She also had to call an ambulance and remain with the patient until the ambulance arrived to transport the patient to the hospital. She goes on to her next patient, a hospice patient and is again delayed because of the need to perform several treatments requested by the physician.

Susan calls her home-care office to report the reason for her two hour delay. The supervisor lightens her patient load so that she can provide quality care and remain healthy herself.

Medical-Surgical Care in a "Business as Usual" Culture

Note that medical-surgical units now care for acute and complex patients who would have been in the ICU 10 years ago.

At 11:00 p.m., a charge nurse discovers that a person that she thought was an RN was an LNA. This scheduling error reduced the unit's licensed staff by one. The oncoming charge nurse feels that another RN is necessary: "We can't even keep everybody alive without another RN." Frantic calls go out to other staff, but none can work because they have already worked many extra shifts. She eventually persuades an evening nurse to stay for the night.

Medical-Surgical Care in a Staff-Friendly Culture

Linda is a medical-surgical nurse on a high-performance team. Everyone has a substantial patient assignment, but, when Linda notices that a patient's vital signs become seriously unstable, she sounds the cardiac arrest code. As Linda works with the code team, Kim, another nurse on the unit, cares for Linda's other patients.

Psychiatric Care in a "Business as Usual" Culture

Sally, a psychiatric RN, remarks to Jen, another RN, "Jen, we're working together on Christmas."

Jen replies, "That's great. I love to work with you."

Sally then corrects Jen's perception. "No. You don't understand. It's only you and I who are scheduled—no one else."

They both know that six staff members are needed for safe care, but, on Christmas Day, Jen and Sally must get by with a staff equivalent of four: two people working 8 hours, with four staff each working 4 hours. No injuries occur, but, with staff so short, there was a greater risk of injury for both patients and staff.

Psychiatric Care in a Staff-Friendly Culture

The 3-to-11 staff on a psychiatric unit requested opportunities for professional growth. Along with the manager, the nurses devise a schedule to cover for each other.

Organizations without a staff-friendly culture fail to realize that negative environments diminish their reputation. Most nurses look at employment ads and immediately eliminate those with poor reputations. Nurses don't apply for positions if they know that the glowing words in the ads are a sham.

Solutions

Use Buzz to Attract Nurses

Nurses, like patients, listen to the buzz about health care facilities. Nurses rely on what they hear from their peers when deciding where to work. They ask their peers about safety issues, staff turnover, and whether they will be treated with respect.

Nurses become skeptical when a facility seems to be replacing most of their staff. If they notice ads for a director of nursing, education director, some supervisory positions, as well as RNs, LPNs, and LNA/CNAs (all shifts, full- and part-time), they wonder why most of the staff has left. Most good nurses steer clear of such facilities.

Some organizations simply do nothing and then hope that the nursing crisis will go away by itself. But the revolving door continues to turn, with nurses coming and going. Money that could be better spent on constructive projects goes out of the door, along with the departing nurses.

View Your Nurses as Assets

Funds for human resources are really an investment in organizational success. High staff turnover reduces the return on that investment. Patients consider nurses as essential assets to their care, but management tends to consider nursing as an expense—a large one. Good managers are taught to maximize assets and minimize expenses. And, because nurses are viewed as an expense, staffing cuts seem to be a logical way to balance the budget. Many organizations have cut their nursing budgets severely.

However, those budget cuts have triggered the nursing shortage and produced burnout and low morale. In some institutions, the quality of nursing care continues to spiral downward, resulting in a vicious cycle of further revenue shortfalls.

According to generally accepted accounting practices (GAAP), an intangible asset is defined as follows: an asset lacking physical substance. The main intangible used in financial statements is "goodwill" (the monetary value of a business's reputation). Although GAAP does not allow companies to list expert employees—nurses or highly trained high-tech employees— as intangible assets in financial documents, expert employees still function as assets. They increase a company's value. Therefore, most high-tech companies value their highly trained employees as assets. Health care organizations should do the same: they should value their nurses as assets.

Document Nursing Value Quantitatively

1. Perform a cost benefit analysis: managers and clinical nurses can justify their requests with a cost benefit analysis. For example, Table 10.1 shows how you can quantify the financial advantages of adding one more nurse.
2. Create a ratio. In this case, for every $1 that you spend to hire an additional nurse, you reap $10 in benefits, which equals a sound business decision. Your cost-to-benefit ratio is 1:10. According to researchers at the University of Minnesota School of Public Health, hiring even one extra nurse can help save lives: "For every 1,000 hospitalized patients, reviewers estimated that adding one full-time RN per patient day could save five patient lives in the intensive care unit, five lives on medical floors, and six surgical patient lives" (Fauntleroy, 2007).
3. Calculate your opportunity costs: You may wonder what the opportunity costs are. Suppose you have $30,000, and decide to buy a car. You could pay $30,000 for your car, or you could buy one for $20,000 and have $10,000 left over. If you decide to buy the $30,000 car, by default, you give up having a less expensive car with $10,000 left over. The alternative that you gave up represents your opportunity costs. In other words, your trade-off was to give up the $10,000 and less expensive car for the higher-priced car.

   What could you have done with the $10,000 that you gave up by buying the more expensive car? You could have opened a savings account, gone on an expensive vacation, or used it for a

Table 10.1

COST BENEFIT ANALYSIS OF NURSE STAFFING			
Cost of adding one full-time equivalent		Benefits of adding one full-time equivalent	
Salary	$51,500	Decreased litigation	$500,00
		Avoid premium pay	$10,000
		Decreased sick time	$5,000
Total costs	$51,500	Total benefits	$515,000

down payment on a house. Those three items—savings account, vacation, and house—represent part of your opportunity costs. They represent the trade-off that you made: an expensive car instead of something else.

How do opportunity costs relate to nursing? Health care organizations have miscalculated their opportunity costs. As described, your opportunity costs are measured by the trade-offs that you make. A common health care trade-off is to save money by using inadequate staffing (short-term solution) and live with the long-term consequences (high turnover).

Another example is that, when you allow an unsatisfactory work environment to continue, by default, you have chosen high nurse turnover and have given up a stable nursing staff. (Managers who delay action to repair negative cultures must live with the long-term result, high staff turnover.)

4. Calculate the cost of nursing turnover, as shown in Table 10.2. As you can see, losing just six nurses costs you $140,000. Your opportunity costs in that situation are that you could have spent the $140,000 on giving 50 nurses 2 weeks off with pay or on providing a 2-week educational sabbatical for 50 nurses.

What about the $390,000 it cost you to lose 10 nurses? You could have used that amount on all of the following:

- A full-time person in charge of solving the root causes of problems ($77,000)
- An educational conference for 30 nurses ($15,000)
- A college course for two nurses ($3,000)
- New computer equipment ($5,000)

Table 10.2

THE COST OF NURSE TURNOVER

	6	10*
Number of nurses leaving per year	6	10*
Cost of orientation	$60,000	$100,000
Cost of premium pay to cover staffing "holes"	$30,000	$70,000
Training associated costs (when productivity is less than 100%)	$30,000	$90,000
Cost of advertising, interview time, sign-on bonus, time to manage short staffing	$20,000	$130,000
Total	**$140,000**	**$390,000**

*Some from Intensive Care Unit and the Operating Room.

- Two extra weeks off with pay for 50 nurses or a 2-week sabbatical for 50 nurses ($140,000)

You could get all of that and still have $150,000 left over.

5.   Raise your return on investment (ROI).

The money you saved by reducing nurse turnover is only the beginning. It gets better. With lower nurse turnover and a staff-friendly culture, quality of care and services improve. Patient safety improves, and risk declines. You avoid expensive litigation that can cost more than $5 million per case.

High patient safety improves your reputation in the community. More physicians and patients want to use your facility. As competent and experienced nurses become familiar with your excellent reputation, they want to work for you. You become the employer of choice for nurses. You have just turned a vicious cycle of decline into a vitalizing cycle of success. Your gross revenue increases.

Plan Your ROI on Nursing

Organizations save money when they decrease nurse turnover. A 300-bed hospital can save roughly $500,000 annually by reducing nurse turnover by a mere 3–5%.

What if you, the manager, could choose the ROI? Would you choose 20% or 30% a year? Why stop? Why not double or triple your money? Human resource investments, particularly in nursing, are an investment on which you choose your own rate of return. You only have to act.

For example, assume that, as the vice president of patient care, you spend $25,000 in a year to educate nurse managers on raising nurse retention: You coach your managers to form solid relationships with their staff (respect each other, act in a trustworthy way, and communicate effectively). You review preferred delegation and decision-making strategies so that your nurses can solve patient problems on the spot, without going up and down a long chain of command.

After the training, the managers of 30-bed units are able to reduce their turnover by 3% over the year. Each unit achieves $50,000 savings in recruitment, orientation, and overtime costs. With six nurse managers, you have created a gross savings of $300,000. Subtracting the $25,000 in training costs gives you a net savings of $275,000. You have just multiplied your investment of $25,000 in management training costs by 11, to a return of $275,000—an 1100% ROI. You have solidly raised the return on your human resource investment. What a wise choice!

Solve Root Problems

When nurses encounter problems in their jobs, they essentially have two choices: solve the immediate problem only, or solve the root cause along with the immediate problem.

The nurses in the Harvard University study (Tucker, Edmonson, & Spear, 2002) described in Chapter 2 used first-order problem solving most of the time. This means that their problems were likely to recur because the cause was never eliminated.

This study indicated that work environment is a critical factor in the success of clinical nurses. What this means to managers is that nurses have to face the same problems happening over and over again without much chance to intervene. It's no wonder that clinical nurses lose their enthusiasm and burn out.

The good news is that these environmental factors are within management control, they are free, and they can be changed easily. Organizations need managers who are willing to identify and solve root problems. How?

- Think about your own experiences. Review your organization's incidents and consider whether some of them could have been avoided if you had identified their root causes.
- Apply some of the suggestions from the Harvard study:

First, if workers are to engage in root cause removal, this activity must be an explicit part of their job and enough time allocated for removal efforts.

Second, there needs to be frequent opportunities for communicating about problems with individuals who are responsible for supplying frontline workers with materials or information . . . There must be convenient opportunities in the course of the day for workers to give feedback.

Third, when the signal is given that there is a problem, proper attention must be paid to it. We must recognize communication as a valid step in the direction of improvement. Often the best that the worker could do was to merely raise the issue, but too often this worker ran the risk of being considered a "complainer." We did not observe any instances where the nurse contacted someone about a trivial or insignificant exception. In fact, we observed several occasions where we were surprised that the nurse did not raise awareness around a problem that we felt could have serious consequences (Tucker, Edmonson, & Spear, 2002).

Nurse Control Over Staffing Levels Help Facilities

Some organizations empower their clinical nurses to make staffing decisions. The managers of these nurses have coached them about their unit's
staffing strategies. As in most patient-care units, the nurses understood
the usual mix of staff for different census levels. But, what was different
was that the clinical nurses had the power to raise or lower the staffing
level based solely on their assessment of patient acuity, staff expertise,
and other "in the moment" factors. The manager and these nurses trust
each other and work together. The nurses have entrepreneurial attitudes
and have a personal stake as if they are personally responsible for the
success of their organization.

The following two examples illustrate the difference between staff
with and without an entrepreneurial attitude.

A 20-bed unit has a census of 19 patients. A referral agency calls asking whether the unit has an available male bed. The nurse without an
entrepreneurial attitude says, "No. We only have a female bed." The nurse
with an entrepreneurial attitude says, "Yes, I will take the admission." She
is willing to do the extra work involved in moving the female patient from
the private room into the empty bed, making room for the male admission. Assuming that the transfer and admission are otherwise appropriate,
the second nurse feels that it is her responsibility to keep the unit full
because it makes her organization more successful.

Relationship Management

Autocratic management styles are still too common in health care.
According to AHRQ data (Agency for Healthcare Research and Quality),
"Nurses cited practice deterrents such as pay inequity (for degree of
responsibilities and skills), lack of respect for hospital nurses, and safety
concerns for themselves and patients. They also voiced concerns about
exhaustion, stress, excessive work demands, and work-related injuries,
increasingly ill patients, mandatory overtime, and nurse shortages. These
problems raised the negative attitudes toward nursing" (AHRQ, 2008).

Some organizations have tried to reverse this trend with shared governance, involving clinical staff participation, sharing power, and avoiding
micromanagement. Micromanagement commonly occurs when managers
still oversee every minor detail after delegating decision-making authority to another. Micromanagement is unpleasant for the delegatee, and
the duplication of effort wastes time and money. Micromanagement also

destroys innovation because staff members are prevented from using their own approach, defeating the purpose of shared governance. This does not mean that managers should abandon their staff after delegation. As a manager, you can still be a good resource person and be available to answer questions, check on progress, and introduce staff to other people who can help.

Reports of micromanagement and bureaucracy in other industries have the same destructive edge as described by research:

> Marion called the person in charge of marketing with a question about something and I promptly got a call from the CEO telling me that's not the way things work. He told me that Marion should have called him and he would have relayed the request to the head of marketing, who'd talk to the proper supervisor in the marketing department, who would talk to the right employee, who would get back to the supervisor, who'd get back to the head of marketing, who'd relay the information to the CEO, who would then call me. (Jennings, 2002)

Looking at groups that are not health care organizations helps us understand our own bureaucratic wastes of time and money. Nurses who have been involved in committees have found that their input can be ignored, resulting in their efforts being just "busy work." Consider the cost of an average committee. Twenty nurses attending meetings for just 1 hour each month costs over $6,000 a year. This is an expensive mistake unless you are willing to listen to your committees.

Nurses become cynical when their reasoned input is disregarded. Discuss your staffing strategies with your nurses so that they are able to support them. Then show nurses that you value their efforts to add value.

Suppose that a cardiac patient's family has had a difficult adjustment to his hospitalization, reacting with underlying anger and fear. As the charge nurse slowly forms a relationship with the family, they ask her to help them solve a problem with the visiting hours. The charge nurse clarifies limits and finalizes a customized plan to meet the needs of the patient and family. This charge nurse has two main accomplishments: better customer service and stronger patient loyalty (thus reducing the patient resentment that often leads to litigation).

When you champion your nurses, you build strong relationships. The best nurse managers insist that the staff be respected. Good managers also enforce the policy, "We don't 'do' rude here," and they support nurses who assertively enforce this philosophy as well.

For example, a physician in a hurry can't find a chart and makes an irate comment to a nearby nurse. She calmly acknowledges his need for the chart but is clearly assertive and explains that his angry comments were not appropriate. She says, "I get frustrated looking for charts too, but it's not okay to take out your anger on me." This nurse knows that her nurse manager will support her even if the physician complains about the limits that she set.

Nurses are knowledge workers, and they constitute an important part of an organization's intellectual capital. Now, intellectual capital is considered one of the organization's most important assets.

Adequate rest for staff is an insurance policy for management success. Even equipment—capital assets—need downtime. How much more important are your human assets? Nurses need time to rest. Review your full-time nurse schedules for the past six months and look for the number of times that each nurse has had a four-day stretch of time off. If your nurses have worked without a minimum of two four-day breaks in the past six months, you are risking staff burnout. Your nurses need enough downtime to recharge their energy.

Assess your responsiveness to nursing needs. Calculate how many staff issues have remained unresolved for 60 days or more. Unresolved issues (frequently unsolved root problems) are one of the major causes of the nursing crisis. Set a 30-day deadline to resolve unresolved issues. Create a critical path to keep you on schedule (Table 10.3). Or delegate your unresolved issues to the clinical nurses involved, along with enough

Table 10.3

CRITICAL PATH

Week 1	Week 2	Week 3	Week 4
Vacation schedule	Talk with staff	Write tentative schedule	Final schedule
Increase charge nurse autonomy, especially for staffing and safety responsibilities	Meet with charge nurses to ask for input	Schedule meeting to coach charge nurses and discuss staffing strategies	Meet with charge nurses to begin new responsibilities, to set up communication channels, and to schedule ongoing opportunities for further discussion

authority for them to implement their solutions. Then support the decisions that your nurses make. Clinical nurses need managers who are willing to create and maintain positive work environments. They need managers who are willing to support them. Clinical nurses need managers who understand nursing's true value. Are you up to the challenge?

Consider using the ANA (American Nursing Association's) staffing guidelines as a practical guide to understanding the big picture of nurse staffing:

> Shifting the nursing paradigm away from an industrial model to a professional model would move the industry and organizations away from the technical approach of measuring time and motion to one that examines myriad aspects of using knowledge workers to provide quality care. This shift would spell the end to the "nurse-is-a-nurse-is-a nurse" mentality by focusing on the complexity of unit activities and level(s) of nurse competency needed to provide quality patient care. (American Nurses Association, 2004)

There are other organizations with a similar approach:

The Robert Wood Johnson Foundation (RWJF) and the American Association of Retired Persons (AARP) Foundation recently announced a joint effort to address the 1.1 million nurse workforce shortage by creating the Center to Champion Nursing in America. Additional information about the Center can be found at www.championnursing.org (Trossman, 2006).

As nursing and business periodicals report, most RNs continue to perceive the shortage as a major problem for early detection of patient complications. Over 75% of RNs perceive the shortage as a major problem for the quality of their own work life and the quality of patient care (Beurhaus, Donelin, Ulrich, Norman, & Dittus, 2005).

Nurse Residency Programs for New Graduates

One approach to reduce the turnover of new graduate nurses is to create residency programs. Residency programs hire new RNs with the understanding that the organization will provide a formalized training program with education and support for up to a year. As the new RNs transition from advanced beginner to competent nurse in the acute-care environment, the nurse resident is not counted in total number of FTEs (full-time equivalent). Some facilities avoid residency programs because of the expense, but others see them as good long-term investments in their staffing commitment.

BEST PRACTICE: HOW A SUPPORTIVE WORK ENVIRONMENT IMPROVES NURSE STAFFING

Diana Halfer MSN, RN, NE-BC, Administrator, Clinical and Organizational Development, "Building Excellence Together", Children's Memorial Medical Center, Chicago, IL

At Children's Memorial Hospital in Chicago, Illinois, our organizational strategy is to drive innovation in employee engagement, retention, and recruitment to achieve workforce needs.

Central to staffing success is the collaboration between nursing and human resource leaders in developing a comprehensive workforce plan during a national nursing shortage.

A key branding strategy has been to provide a supportive work environment in order to become a top employer.

- The evidence is clear about the bottom-line impact of being a top employer.
- Top employers are leaders in their industry sector.
- The hallmarks of a supportive work environment are when employees:
  - Trust their leaders
  - Feel pride in their work
  - Enjoy their coworkers.

The Children's Memorial leadership vision is to provide a supportive work environment, in order to improve retention and engagement and to be recognized as a top employer in order to improve recruitment.

- This vision demonstrates commitment in a dramatic way and has received an enthusiastic employee response in helping the hospital become a better place to work.

To accomplish the vision, we have made a promise to all employees.
The Employer Promise:

- Support both personal and professional goals
- Provide a challenging but compassionate work environment
- Recognize strong performance
- Listen to and act on employee feedback.

The promise has been used to assess human resource practices, address gaps, and develop programs and policies to make the promise real.

The outcomes for nursing have been visible in satisfaction and retention. In 2007, overall employee and physician satisfaction survey results were at the 97th percentile, nursing satisfaction far exceeded national norms (5.89 versus the national norm of 4.55), and 82% of the nurses rated the employment experience as a 6 ("like it a lot") or a 7 ("love it"). The hospital-wide focus of having a supportive work environment has produced low rates of nursing turnover (7.2%) and vacancy (5.6%) during a national nursing shortage.

Core organizational competencies further define the work culture needed for success: teamwork, service excellence, and innovation.

Feedback—from patients and families, employees, and physicians—is regularly collected via surveys, focus groups, leadership rounds, and town hall meetings.

Leaders respond with focused interventions, avoiding "boiling the ocean," to sustain momentum on the vital few tactics that make a difference in the employee work experience.

Organizational strengths identified in 2007 were employee satisfaction survey feedback, which identified many areas of strengths:

- The hospital was viewed as a great place to work.
- Pride existed in the mission, quality of care, and teamwork.
- Benefits were viewed as outstanding.
- Professional development opportunities were appreciated.

Feedback for improvement targeted tenacious issues: high span of control for managers, resulting in pockets of individuals who did not work well together. Acting on the feedback, leaders focused on hiring for cultural fit, holding employees accountable for teamwork behaviors, addressing the span of control issues, and accelerating physician integration into the culture

Selection of new employees includes the following:

- Behaviorally based interview questions are used to select new employees who will fit with the organizational cultural values of teamwork, service, strong work ethic, and ability to work in a fast-paced environment.
- Leaders proactively recruit when there are no position vacancies. Candidates with a good résumé or a great referral are interviewed even when there is not an available position.

■ Leaders communicate carefully with strong second-position choices so that, if another opening occurs, the candidate has a favorable impression of the organization.

Integral to the promise is recognizing strong performance in teamwork and service excellence behaviors. Peers nominate and select exceptional employee, nurse, physicians, and teams for awards: the Julia Porter Outstanding Employee Award, the A. Todd Davis Outstanding Physician Award, and the Earl J. Frederick Outstanding Team Award. Nurses are recognized throughout the year: the American Nursing Credentialing Center's Certified Nurse Day, the Daisy Award, Nurses' Week, Nursing Exemplar Award, and Nursing Preceptor Month. Celebrations are held for recipients of internal grant awards for innovation, through the Prince Charitable Trust Nursing Scholar and Sabbatical Programs, and for research, through the Walter W. and Jean Young Shaw Research in Nursing and Allied Health Program.

Strong performance is rewarded through an annual merit compensation program and employee results sharing, which pays out when service excellence and financial goals are met. The clinical advancement program for nurses was used as a model for similar programs for respiratory therapists and medical-imaging technologists. Expert clinical work is rewarded with a promotional bonus on advancement and an annual bonus with active participation in hospital goals.

Professional development opportunities contribute to job satisfaction and retention. Career development is fostered through a new graduate-nurse mentoring program, clinical skills certification courses, guest lectureships, advanced practice-nursing grand rounds, funding support for conference attendance and nursing specialty certifications, and innovation and research grants. On-site college courses and an MBA curriculum are funded through a tuition reimbursement program.

To support nurses working in a challenging work environment, Children's Memorial was one of 13 pilot hospitals participating in Transforming Care at the Bedside, a program funded by the Robert Wood Johnson Foundation in partnership with the Institute for Health Care Improvement. Inpatient nurses led tests of change in order to improve the quality of care. Examples include a proactive health and wellness program, a morning staffing huddle to increase patient safety awareness, and daily quiet time, using an Ear Noise Meter to increase awareness of environmental noise for pediatric patients.

External recognition for Children's Memorial has produced free marketing through media attention and publications from American Nurses

Credentialing Center, Health Care Advisory Board, *Working Mother's Magazine*, and the *Chicago Magazine*. An early adopter of the Magnet standards, Children's Memorial became the first free-standing children's hospital to become designated Magnet in 2001, and it has been recognized by the Health Care Advisory Board as one of five "Destination Nursing Organizations" in the nation. Designation by *Working Mother's Magazine* as a 100 Best Company and the *Chicago Magazine* as one of the top 25 places to work promotes the branding strategy.

Promoting Smart Staffing

TIPS FOR CLINICAL NURSES

- Keep a healthy balance between life and work.
- Think long term.
- Value your work.
- Be patient.
- Support management's positive staffing efforts.

TIPS FOR MANAGERS

- Avoid mandatory overtime.
- Use stable staffing to increase patient satisfaction.
- Motivate; don't coerce.
- Hire for attitude and train for skills.
- Utilize the intuition of nurses.

TIPS FOR EDUCATORS

- Teach students how to be good at coaching.
- Include problem-solving strategies in your curriculum.
- Be honest about staffing issues.
- Maintain your own clinical skills.
- Avoid defensiveness.

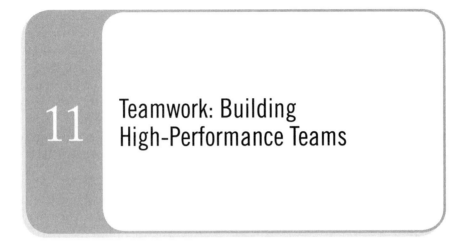

11 Teamwork: Building High-Performance Teams

If teams learn, they become a microcosm for learning throughout the organization. —*Peter M. Senge*

Use teamwork to address the following health care issues:

- Managers continue having difficulty staffing their facilities because of increased demand for health care services and decreased supplies of nurses.
- Workloads for nurses and other health care workers continue to increase.
- Medical errors continue at a high rate.
- Baby Boomer health care requirements raise the demand for additional services. Baby Boomers are educated, articulate, and assertive and do not allow their needs to be put off with weak platitudes.
- The bottom line of many health care organizations continues running in the red in direct proportion to the high costs of finding and retaining competent staff.
- Organizations need the efficiency and financial savings that high-performance teams offer.

A serious obstacle to high-performance teams is the attitude of "every nurse for herself." This attitude has proliferated for various reasons. Authoritarian and coercive management styles have resulted in dysfunctional cultures that block cooperative efforts. But nurses themselves have often returned to adolescent behavior styles, focusing on rejection and pitting one staff member against another.

Nurses need positive cultures and high-performance teams so that they can work smarter, not just faster. Instituting high-performance teams costs nothing; the key factor is attitude—of staff members and management alike.

In my experience, I have found that high-performance teams raise productivity without increasing either medical errors or nurse burnout. Because health care is labor-intensive, this higher productivity also reduces costs.

Consider a typical day on a high-performance team:

> The nurses arrive for work. They don't object to heavy assignments because they know that others will help them if their workload becomes unmanageable. Patient-care units are unpredictable because most patients are medically complex and unstable. One nurse caring for five patients may have to manage several medical emergencies at the same time. Staff members can manage these emergencies better when everyone works cooperatively.
>
> High-performance team members value diversity and ask each other for advice. Mutual respect builds commitment to the team and results in everyone's accomplishing more. Everyone pitches in when three admissions arrive during a 2-hour period. While the RN is assessing the patients, the secretary or LNA/CNA orients the patients to the unit and the LNA/CNA helps the secretary assemble the charts. Later, the secretary may be swamped with orders. The RN notes extra orders or enters them into the computer. They all work as hard as they can, no matter whose job it is.
>
> In the end, the workload evens out fairly. Staff members remember how others helped them when they were the busy ones. They joke with their colleagues to manage stress. As they leave work, they say, "I can hardly believe how much we were able to accomplish today." They feel pride and gratitude for the team that helped them accomplish so much. They were able to accomplish more with less effort.

High-performance teams also prepare units to manage unexpected staffing problems. Consider the following example:

> All of the licensed nursing staff on one shift were sick for a week, except for one RN and one LPN. The RN was able to manage the unit with less

nursing staff by delegating things in a different way. Within legal limitations, certain parts of the admission process and other work usually assigned to nursing staff were delegated to LNA/CNAs. This certainly was not an optimal situation, but it helped them survive a temporary staffing shortage and gave them flexibility without sacrificing quality.

Is this situation a fantasy? No. This scenario is a composite of the day-to-day experiences of nurses working on high-performance teams. Team members use humor to decrease stress and create a relaxed working environment and positive atmosphere for patients, who would sometimes comment, "We love it when the nurses laugh with each other." They are also able to model stress management techniques.

The foundation of high-performance teams is a web of positive relationships that are built over time. The manager often initiates these relationships, and the resulting trust that staff members have in their manager enables a feeling of security to envelop everyone. Staff members, confident in their roles, are able to raise patient satisfaction and contribute to their organization's bottom line.

Staff meetings are important; knowing that their opinions are valued, most of the team members attend them. When a staff member contributes a good idea, the manager implements that idea in days, not months. Good managers know that the finest ideas come from direct-care staff who notice ways to improve their workplace. Staff members are motivated to keep their ideas flowing because they get satisfaction from seeing their ideas put into practice. They know that they also have a better work environment.

When a manager wants to fill staffing holes, team members cooperate and often volunteer to rearrange their schedules to fill vacancies. They know that, when they need time off, their manager will at least put forth a good effort to accommodate them.

The Smart Nursing Process for Building High-Performance Teams

1. Form relationships.

   Do you want all your nurses to be cookie-cutter nurses, all the same? One secret to building relationships is to encourage employees to be themselves. It is exhausting to have to keep up a false front. Get to know your nurses' true identities, and show them your own true self. Of course, no one is perfect, but the strengths and weaknesses of individual team members counterbalance each other. The connections between team members can become your greatest strength.

2. Empower your staff.

Nurses need power if you expect them to strive for excellence. A nurse's intuition, honed by many years of education and experience, suggests the right action. Many nurses say intuition is responsible for their most astute decisions. This is how experienced nurses add value to your organization.

Empowered nurses avoid burnout because they control the quality of the care that they provide. Psychological principles maintain that people experience reduced stress when they retain control of a situation, even if the situation is negative. And patients are grateful to have such strong advocates working on their behalf.

3. Choose smart strategies.

Your staff members need to understand senior management's perspective in order to work toward organizational success. But many organizations build their strategic plans and then keep them at the board level, far away from the people who are responsible for making them succeed. That is why they fail. Plans must be living breathing undertakings. When employees understand your plan, they are able to collaborate and strengthen your whole organization.

Many CEOs sincerely value contributions from all levels of their staff. But some senior managers only value what their managers do. They fail to recognize that it is the employees who make managers successful. Good managers know that they can succeed only with plenty of dedicated employees on their team.

4. Remove obstacles.

Take the quiz at the end of this chapter to see where you stand on the teamwork continuum. Ask your team members to identify what they think is holding your team back. Ask outside observers for their opinion. Consult with senior management for their advice. Read books on teamwork and learn from the experiences of others. Network with other facilities to see what works for them.

Prioritize your obstacles and take action to remove them; don't just continue to analyze.

5. Give feedback.

Feedback is a gift, a personal and professional gift, so that you can become the best person and have the best team possible. As with any gift, it means more when given with a spirit of generosity and support. Even if the motive is less altruistic, pay attention and evaluate the suggestions objectively. If the feedback seems accurate, incorporate the suggestions into your work.

BEST PRACTICE: A WHOLE SYSTEM'S APPROACH TO TEAMBUILDING

Beth Boynton, RN, MS, Nurse Trainer, Coach, Consultant, Speaker, York Beach, ME

Consider using a Whole System's Approach to teambuilding if difficult dynamics are interfering with productivity. It involves an assessment, feedback loop, creating a safe environment, commitment for change, and focused work.

Assessment: Input regarding concerns, goals, and teambuilding history from leadership and every team member.

Feedback loop: Results of interviews with stakeholders.

Create a safe environment: Facilitated development of team norms, ensuring that respectful communication is standard operating procedure.

Commitment for change: Clear vision, mission, goals, and expectations, with opportunity for all members to express investment.

Focused work: Workshops to build trust and address education needs that have surfaced.

Suggestions for Team Leaders

1. Delegate decision making.

The best managers enable their nurses to solve patient problems on the spot, instead of requiring them to go up and down long chains of command. Delegation promotes patient satisfaction and reduces costs.

Patients become dissatisfied when they are forced to wait while their nurses obtain permission to respond to their needs.

Managers who empower their staff members enjoy higher staff competence.

Managers can use the time saved to build the kind of relationships that improve nurse retention. These relationships are the basis for renewed commitment of their staff members.

2. Coach your staff.

Remember the adage, "Give a man a fish and you feed him for a day; teach him how to fish and you feed him for a lifetime." Maximize your staff's expertise with coaching.

Coach your staff members to make good decisions, instead of telling them what to do. Coaching and granting autonomy complement each other because they both access the essence of your employees' greatest strengths.

Coaching creates a path for your employees' ideas to flow. Diverse viewpoints contribute to your success. Managers lose these contributions when staff members are expected to be replicas of one another.

3. Think long term.

Results don't happen overnight. Coaching is an investment that takes time and patience, but corporate results grow quickly when employees are able to contribute their best ideas.

Coaching is a long-term process. Staff members need clear, consistent communication and support over a period of time before they understand how to use their best ideas at work.

4. Encourage lifelong learning.

Hire for attitude; train for skills. You leap ahead of health care change when your staff members have lifelong learning habits. Because each employee has different interests, your collective employee intelligence is comprehensive and is an asset to your organization.

Managers can promote lifelong learning by encouraging their employees to have curious minds, to think before acting, and to verbalize their interests and concerns.

5. Be a good role model.

You are more likely to achieve results when you influence your staff by setting an example. If you want to be respected, respect others. If you want your staff to be lifelong learners, be one yourself. The same goes for courtesy, autonomy, and other desired staff attributes.

Productivity and quality gains will reward you.

Suggestions for Team Members

1. Value diversity.

   In his book *From Conflict to Creativity* (2001), Sy Landau reveals how to unleash creativity and enhance productivity with or without existing conflict. Health care needs this approach. At times, health care employees spend so much time and energy attacking each other and dealing with the resulting chaos that there is little time left to accomplish any work.

2. Think critically.

   Be confident and think for yourself. Good organizations support professionals who use common sense when applying policies and procedures. Professionals are most valuable when they come up with simple, cost-effective solutions that are focused on solving patient problems.

3. Cross-train.

   It doesn't make sense to have too many staff on one unit and too few on another. Patient census and acuity change rapidly. Cross-training improves your organization's ability to manage those changes. However, staff members may need to set necessary limits so that others do not exploit their flexibility. Organizations should both train and reward staff for broadening their skills.

4. Use synergy.

   Synergy occurs when a group achieves more together than the sum of what the group members could have accomplished individually. Some examples of synergy are brainstorming, helping a peer with a difficult admission, or creating an education program for the entire team.

   Creating more from less is a good approach while attempting to cope with rising staff shortages and decreasing revenue. Staff members prefer to be productive. The obstacles that hold them back frustrate staff more than anyone else.

5. Build your own self-esteem.

   Low self-esteem magnifies the imperfections of others. Successful people focus on maximizing their own strengths instead of criticizing those of others. Because the skill mix within the team is complementary, individual weaknesses matter less. And teaching each other is a common team practice that helps individuals become stronger professionals.

Every manager and clinical nurse devises his or her own way to add high-performance teams to the staffing strategy. Customization is a good way is make sure that your high-performance team meets your patients' needs. Many approaches succeed if you adopt the basic principles of respect, dignity, and creativity.

High-performance teams help you achieve the following:

- Manage heavy workloads by allowing nurses to accomplish more with less energy.
- Experience synergy, whereby everyone accomplishes more.
- Raise the value of your most important asset: intellectual capital— the hearts and minds of your employees.
- Raise productivity in a cost-effective way.
- Promote accountability, profitability, and staff retention.
- Increase the effectiveness of your strategic plan.
- View all sides of issues, using peers with diverse perspectives as advisors.
- Make better decisions with quality input from others, allowing them to actually become smarter.
- Recognize opportunities within your problems.
- Encourage staff members to turn conflict into creative solutions.

QUIZ

Do You Work on a High-Performance Team?

Give yourself 1 point for each YES answer.

Questions for Clinical Staff

1. Does your work group produce quality care?
2. Is each person accountable for his or her results?
3. Do you feel authentic at work, or are you expected to play a role?
4. Is communication between staff members effective?
5. Is your group productive?
6. Have you eliminated gripe sessions at work?
7. Are you as happy about the success of others as you are about your own success?

8. Do you have fun?
9. Does your group enjoy positive relationships?
10. Do you have positive attitudes?
11. Are you energized by your work?
12. Do staff members innovate and improve your workplace?
13. Are your peers mutually respectful?
14. Do staff members share important information with others instead of hoarding it?
15. Do staff members have an entrepreneurial approach to their job? That is, do they feel as if their organization's success is directly related to the job that they do?

Questions for Managers

1. When choosing a new staff member, do you consider how she or he will function on your team?
2. Are staff members able to solve employee disputes themselves, or do you have to intervene?
3. Are you a good leader as well as a good manager? ("Leaders do the right things; managers do things right" —Warren Bemis.)
4. Do you discuss staffing goals with your nurses and then give them autonomy to modify staffing levels as needed?
5. Have you implemented at least 95% of your staff members' suggestions within 30 days?
6. Do you insist on respectful behavior from everyone, no matter what his or her position is?
7. Is your staff productive?
8. Is your nursing turnover less than 5%?
9. Is your rate of medical errors low?
10. Do you focus more effort on long-term planning than on managing crises?
11. Is your sense of humor a vital part of your management style?
12. Are your staff meetings well attended?
13. Are you open to diverse opinions from your staff?
14. Are you a good role model?
15. Do you use mandatory overtime for fewer than five shifts per month?

Scoring

(For each quiz)
Score 13–15: Give everyone a pat on the back.

10–12: You are on your way.

7–9: You have the right idea.

4–6: Have a talk with your team members.

0–3: Seek out a great team and ask questions.

Promoting Teamwork

Our current health care environment needs sensible ways to improve productivity. High-performance teams can help. Try them.

TIPS FOR CLINICAL NURSES

- Develop your communication skills.
- Use your intuition.
- Manage conflict constructively.
- Be a lifelong learner.
- Learn from your peers.

TIPS FOR MANAGERS

- Be trustworthy.
- Listen to your staff's suggestions.
- Calculate your team's value.
- Explain how staff can help with your strategic plan.
- Be a coach.

TIPS FOR EDUCATORS

- Use a team approach from the start.
- Develop a curious mind.
- Have a long-term plan.
- Learn critical thinking.
- Ask experienced nurses for teamwork tips.

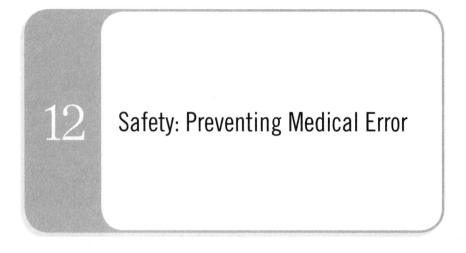

12 Safety: Preventing Medical Error

The foundation of a culture of safety is trust. *—Julianne Morath*

Pick up a newspaper or magazine, watch TV, or talk with a friend; you will hear concerns about patient safety. Visit the National Institute of Health Web site (www.nih.gov) for data about the influence of nurse staffing on patient safety. Many public opinion surveys can be found at the Kaiser Family Foundation site (www.kff.org.), such as the results of a 2004 telephone survey where nearly half (48 %) of adults say they are concerned about health care safety, and over half (55 %) say that they are currently dissatisfied with health care quality in this country (www.kff.org, accessed July 2008).

Risk Management

Nurses As Frontline Risk Managers

Medical errors cause heartaches for patients, their families, and health care professionals. Nurses have the potential to improve patient safety by functioning as frontline risk managers. Because clinical nurses are often the first to notice potential errors, it makes sense to empower nurses to stop errors in time to prevent injury.

Nurses play a crucial role in intercepting medication errors. A study by the IOM found that nurses intercepted 86% of errors made by physicians, pharmacists, and others. The cochairpersons, Kathleen Stevens (EdD, RN, FAAN) and Linda R. Cronenwett (PhD, RN, FAAN) agree that a systems approach is needed to tackle this issue because nurses are often the last line of defense in preventing medication errors (Trossman, 2006).

Nurses try to do as much as they can to protect patients in individual situations, but rarely do they have the power to change the system in order to prevent errors from recurring. For example, a medication nurse notices a dropper bottle in the medication room, picks it up, and notices that the label says "hemoccult developer solution" (a lab test chemical). She recalls an article in a nursing journal describing a tragic medication error when a nurse accidentally put hemoccult developer instead of eye drops into a patient's eyes, causing total blindness. The nurse quickly moved the hemoccult developer to the utility room, but the "near-miss" was never investigated. As a result, the risk level for this organization went up, and it grew every time that managers routinely ignored nursing input.

The Effect of Workarounds on Patient Safety

Workarounds are quite common in health care and can cause medical errors. A workaround is a practice by nurses and others that circumvents an important safety practice—for example, when nurses are supposed to scan the bar code on a patient's identification bracelet but find it easier to use a copy of the patient's bar code and scan that instead. The reason for the safety standard is to ensure that the nurse has the right patient; scanning the duplicate bar code defeats the purpose of the safety standard.

A NURSE SAVED MY LIFE

Terry is a Yale graduate and served as a navigator in World War II [. . .] Looking back on those life and death moments, Terry quietly says, "A nurse saved my life. She was keeping a close watch on me and saw that I was in distress. She called the code and they resuscitated me [. . .] She caught me in time [. . .] This is why I have such a high regard for the nursing profession. If I were in the hospital today, with nurses overworked, I don't know if I would be so fortunate" (Gibson, 2003).

The reason for workarounds is that they overcome a time bottleneck problem. For instance, the identification bracelet bar code is sometimes difficult to scan because it curves around the wrist; thus the workaround.

The solution to workarounds is to make sure that safety standards are easy for nurses to manage in actual practice and to have a high enough staffing level so that nurses have enough time to maintain safety standards exactly as they were intended.

Preventing Medical Errors

Smart Nursing core values and guiding principles of smart health care management help facilities improve patient safety by improving the way that nurses are managed. Understanding that patient safety rates are partly within management control casts a different light on patient safety accountability.

The key to improving patient safety is culture. When organizations maintain cultures of safety, staff members understand that safety is more important than the ego or convenience of anyone—any manager, physician, or staff member.

Safety is more important than the ego or convenience of anyone.

Measure how close you come to a culture of safety with "two highly validated and widely used instruments":

1. The Institute for Health Care Improvement safety climate survey from the Center of Excellence for Patient Safety Research and Practice (2004).
2. The Agency for Health Care Research and Quality (AHRQ) hospital survey on patient safety culture (2006).

Both documents can be downloaded free of charge. (See Smetzer & Navarra, 2007.)

Steps that clinical nurses themselves can take to make drug administration safer can be found at http://newton.nap.edu/catalog/11623 .html3toc, for the complete report ("Preventing Medication Errors—Quality Chasm Series") and at www.iom.edu/CMS/3809/22526/35939/35 943.aspx, for a summary ("Report Brief, Preventing Medication Errors") (*American Nurse Today*, 2006).

Nurse-Physician Collaboration

Nurse-physician collaboration on safety issues is so easy, but it is not always found in practice. Suppose that a physician orders a large dose of a medication with a side effect of lowering blood pressure. Because the nurse knows that this patient's blood pressure has been in the low to normal range, she alerts the physician and expresses her concern that administering this medication may cause this patient's blood pressure to drop too low. The physician expresses his appreciation for the nurse's input and changes the medication order.

CEO Influence on Safety

CEOs are the ones in organizations who set the standard for every single employee. In my experience, the safest organizations all have had one common trait—excellent CEOs. Each time, the CEO has been a positive role model. He or she was held in high esteem by the staff, and there was genuine trust between the CEO and staff. The CEO's actions raised staff morale and built commitment.

Use Smart Nursing to Solve Systems Problems

Many managers continue to overburden their nurses with increasingly heavy clinical tasks. This requires nurses to work faster and faster, instead of allowing them to work smarter.

Managers could raise nurse productivity by adopting Smart Nursing core values and the 10 guiding principles of smart health care management. They could then solve root problems, instead of focusing mainly on the symptoms of problems. If nurses must work in inadequate systems, they lose productivity and accuracy, and they become overtired. If managers listen to frontline nurses, they can identify and solve systems problems, thereby increasing accuracy and reducing nurse fatigue.

Take this example into account. The following responsibilities were the expectations of day-shift RNs during their first hour of work:

1. Listen to report.
2. Assess vital signs for all.
3. Prepare preoperative outpatients for surgery.

4. Pour and administer the morning medications.
5. Provide morning physical care.
6. Supervise breakfast.

Because it was impossible to perform that much work in such a short time, the nurses frequently skipped listening to the report so that they could finish the rest of their tasks. This placed the organization at risk for serious errors. The following example describes the errors that can occur when nurses don't have enough time to listen to report:

A nurse starts to take vital signs without listening to the report. She approaches a patient who is sitting in a chair outside his room. His name band confirms his identity. The nurse takes his blood pressure, uneventfully. It is only later, after listening to the report, that she discovers the patient had a dialysis access catheter inserted in his chest and that he should not have blood pressures taken in one arm. Although taking the blood pressure caused no harm this time, the potential for error was there. Listening to the report is necessary for safety, even in the case of simple procedures such as vital sign assessment.

The nurse manager correctly recognized this situation as a systems problem. Instead of asking nurses to work harder and faster, she consulted with them and reconfigured some of the tasks: Taking vital signs and performing morning care were reassigned to the night-shift LNA/CNAs, and outpatient surgeries were assigned to another unit.

The 7-to-3 RNs were then able to perform their work safely and with excellence. Nursing input had enabled the manager to change a flawed system, allowing the nurses to work safer and smarter.

Tool Kits for Safer Health Care Practices

The AHRQ developed 17 tool kits designed by experts who specialize in patient safety research. They are free and publically available. They range from checklists for medication reconciliation to communication ideas for caregivers. These tool kits also correlate with the National Patient Safety Goals of the Joint Commission. For information and a complete listing of the 17 tool kits, visit http://www.ahrq.gov/qual/pips/ (Hughes, 2008).

How to Identify and Solve Systems Problems

■ Track medical errors and then identify the root causes. Remember to take action to eliminate the root causes of problems so that they don't keep recurring.

■ Track near-misses. Use near-miss reports to identify high-risk issues. Identify the root causes of the near-misses and take action, just as you did for medical errors.

■ Maintain a nonpunitive attitude regarding errors. This enables you to obtain the necessary data to use in preventing future errors.

Create a "Just Culture"

A just culture is one where people can report mistakes, errors, or waste without reprisal or personal risk. This does not mean that individuals are not held accountable for their actions, but it does mean that people are not held responsible for flawed systems in which dedicated and trained people can still make mistakes. A just culture that promotes sharing and disclosure is a precondition for using "lean" because "lean" organizations depend heavily on frontline staff to drive improvements. All staff must feel empowered to identify errors, defects, and systems failures that could lead to an unsafe environment for patients.

The following is paraphrased from Vogelsmeier: The just-culture movement may not work as well for long-term health care organizations as it seems to work for acute health care organizations.

In a study funded by the AHRQ, Jill Scott-Cawiezell found that nursing homes often have punitive reporting systems for medical errors: "Staff perception of fear coupled with the reality that leaders do not protect staff when negative consequences occur [and] that state surveyors are seeking evidence of individual disciplinary action when untoward events occur [or that] potential criminal action may be taken when an individual is involved in a medical error" (Vogelsmeier, 2007).

Some health care organizations categorize errors into three types and respond to the staff member in one of three ways:

■ For the occasional human error, they support the suffering staff member.

■ For carelessness in nursing practice, they provide education so that the nurse will become more careful in practice.

■ For recklessness practice, these organizations reprimand the staff member.

As more health care organizations use "just culture" for longer periods of time, much more information will be available. Network with other nurses and managers to keep up with current developments in just cultures.

Another organization that is a good resource for patient safety and those dealing with medical errors is MITSS, Medically Induced Trauma Support Services Inc. (www.mitss.org), a nonprofit organization, founded in June 2002, whose mission is "To Support Healing and Restore Hope" to patients, families, and clinicians who have been affected by an adverse medical event. Visit their Web site to review the information that is available for patients, staff, and organizations.

Empowerment

Empowering frontline employees enables nurses to become strong patient advocates. Patient symptoms are acted on the first time when a nurse reports a concern, not after a patient's condition has deteriorated. Empowered nurses are in a good position to prevent patient injury, and they receive support for their decisions by their nurse managers.

An example is an empowered nurse who has the authority to prevent inappropriate patient admissions. Patient transfers are often attempted when they do not meet admission criteria. For example, psychiatric patients need medical clearance because mental health units have only a minimal supply of medical equipment. Patients remain safer when they receive care on a properly equipped unit.

Empowering nurses enables managers to use a proactive approach. Sometimes, managers of facilities cut corners thinking that they will be lucky. They hope that tragedy in the form of medical errors will not happen to them. But negative consequences follow poor decisions, and serious errors do occur unless you follow precise safety guidelines. If you continually ignore safety protocols, it is only a matter of time before your facility will experience serious medical errors.

- Be proactive. Staff your units safely.
- Be proactive. Investigate near misses.
- Be proactive. Review and scrutinize the habits of physicians and other professionals with patterns of numerous errors.
- Be proactive. Solve root problems before patients are injured.
- Be proactive. Choose safe, long-term solutions over risky quick fixes.

- Be proactive. Manage with integrity, instead of spending time and energy on expensive cover-ups.
- Be proactive. Design and test safety protocols for results.
- Be proactive. Listen to your clinical staff.

All of these suggestions are within your control, and all of them are free. These suggestions improve patient safety, and you have no excuse to ignore them.

Educating About Safety

Our country's high rate of medical errors endangers patients, organizations, and nurses. What everyone doesn't realize is that it is possible to use education to reduce medical errors while still maintaining high productivity standards.

Use the following suggestions to educate yourself. It is important to look at safety in a holistic way and to demonstrate an intuitive grasp of potentially unsafe situations.

1. Maximize your orientation. Orientation is a time when nurses have an especially high risk of making errors. Take your time. Ask questions, and focus on developing solid safety habits. Orientation is an opportunity to learn as much as you can before being counted as an FTE (full-time equivalent). Use the time wisely.

2. When it seems that you have to respond to many urgent demands at the same time, take that extra second to clear your mind, relax, and take a deep breath—no matter how busy you are. You will find that you are able to complete your work safely and on time.

3. Use positive self-talk. Say to yourself, "I will work quickly, but not so quickly as to make errors. I don't want to rush this treatment and cause heartaches to my patient and myself."

4. Always check medication labels three times! Yes! Three times every time! Experienced nurses with good safety records find their own errors before giving the medications. For example, after carefully retrieving a medication, during the second check, they may discover that the medication is wrong. They are then able to replace the medication with the appropriate one.

Nurses also find that their fast-paced environments can be distracting, but they can correct their errors on the second or third check before administering a medication to the patient.

5. Always ask yourself the "Five Rights": right medication, right dose, right time, right route, and right patient.
6. Use at least two patient identifiers whenever taking blood samples or administering medications or blood products.
7. Look up unfamiliar medications in reference books.
8. Pay attention to your intuition when something seems wrong.
9. Inquire about questionable situations before you administer the medication.

As these safety rules become automatic, you will find that you can work just as fast with rules as without them. Don't ever cut corners on safety practices to save time.

The application of Smart Nursing core values and guiding principles is cost-effective, and it promotes safety with accountability, respect, and empowerment. But any system is only as strong as the staff members who carry out the safety protocols. No protocol can replace the value of a competent and caring staff who skillfully ensure that the protocols produce the best results possible.

Almost 50% of the Joint Commission's standards are directly related to safety. *Improving America's Hospitals* is the Joint Commission's annual report on quality and safety, with performance measures and safety goals. The Joint Commission has also created The Speak-Up Initiatives, a national program to urge patients to take a more active role in preventing health care errors.

Two Evidence-Based Patient Safety Resources

1. A comprehensive resource, *Patient Safety and Quality: An Evidence-Based Handbook for Nurses*, is a 1,400-page document, released in April 2008, with 89 contributors representing a broad range of researchers. You can download individual chapters or the entire document at www.ahrq.gov (Hughes, 2008). This resource also has many attached articles listed for further reading and allows you to examine the research details on which the report is based. If you need research regarding patient safety, this report could save you from having to find the articles individually.

Some themes for review in this report are the following:

- "A systems approach to patient safety and the impact of leadership and communication on the safety process" (Hughes, 2008).
- Critical safety systems embedded in each level of the system [interdisciplinary] (Hughes, 2008; AHRQ, 2008).
- An informed culture of safety:
  - Bidirectional communication is open and honest.
  - Trust exists at all levels of the organization.
  - Messengers are trained and rewarded for improving systems.
  - The system is just in the treatment of employees; reporting of errors is valued.
  - Lifelong learning from mishaps is identified and appreciated (Hughes, 2008; AHRQ, 2008).

2. In 2006, the National Quality Forum (NQF) updated its report, *Safe Practices for Better Health Care*, creating a list of 30 safe practices that should be universally utilized. One of the NQF recommendations is that "governance boards and senior administrative leaders take accountability for reducing patient safety risks related to nurse staffing decisions and the provision of financial resources for nursing services." (National Quality Forum)

The Lucian Leape Institute at the National Patient Safety Foundation (www.npsf.org) is an independent nonprofit organization that has been pursuing one mission—improving the safety of patients and supporting the many efforts already underway within the health care field. It is an important resource for nurses interested in patient safety.

The Effect of Communication on Safety

Many of the recommendations of the Joint Commission, the NQF, and the Patient Safety Foundation depend on communication. Internal and external strategies (Morath, 2004) to create safe spaces to talk about safety, to promote information sharing, and to create systems that promote a culture of safety include the following:

- Focus groups
- Executive rounds
- Mini-courses

- Safety action teams
- Dialogues

BEST PRACTICE: HOW WE ARE BUILDING OUR CULTURE OF SAFETY

Patricia Byrnes Schmehl, Administrator, Women's Services, Inova Fairfax Hospital Women's Center, Falls Church, VA

Our Obstetrics and Gynecology Department started working to improve our culture of safety in response to leadership concerns about focusing more on reactive responses to errors than on proactive error prevention. We hoped to reduce actual errors and reverse this situation. We wanted to manage all of the safety data in a timely manner by setting aside a regular time to develop prevention strategies.

We created a team called the Women's Common Cause Analysis (CCA) that meets weekly to manage all patient safety information. Core members of the Women's CCA meeting are the Department Chairman, Senior Director of Women's Services, Director, Project Management, Clinical Specialist, and Quality, and Risk Management. In addition to this core group, physicians, residents, directors, and safety coaches are invited to attend on a rotating basis.

This meeting provides a safe environment for staff to identify ways to improve the safety of patients and staff. The purpose of this group includes the following:

1. To review safety data from various sources (occurrence reports, mislabeled specimens, red rule violations, targeted audits, and anecdotal information).
2. To address immediate concerns.
3. To identify trends and concerns.
4. To develop a safety message or "safety huddle"—based on the risks that we have identified—that is shared with all staff.

We use the safety huddle to communicate information from the Women's CCA meeting and as an opportunity to dialogue with staff about our message, to solicit staff safety concerns, and to learn about the staff's "good catches." This safety huddle is led by the Department Director. In addition to sharing the message for the week, a specific topic is addressed for feedback and is sent back to the team for consideration.

Promoting Safety

TIPS FOR CLINICAL NURSES

- Be firm about safety issues.
- Clear your mind when you have multiple issues happening at once.
- Be holistic about safety issues.
- Use positive self-talk to pace yourself.
- Listen to patient's concerns about safety.

TIPS FOR MANAGERS

- Empower nurses to make safety decisions.
- Be proactive.
- Build interdisciplinary approaches to safety.
- Create a learning organization.
- Document near-misses.

TIPS FOR EDUCATORS

- Encourage nurses to develop an entrepreneurial attitude.
- Encourage your students to have intellectual curiosity.
- Explore health care power issues.
- Teach nurses to be risk managers.
- Encourage students to participate in safety improvement strategies.

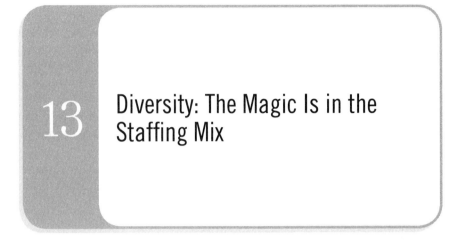

13 Diversity: The Magic Is in the Staffing Mix

We can derive strength from our human bonds rather than building walls out of human differences.   *—Max DePree*

People are different. Diversity in the area of health care could be our greatest strength if we embraced diversity instead of rebuking it. Individual variance causes unnecessary conflict when differences are considered threats. In this chapter, we use the term *diversity* to mean differences of all types—in personality, skills, outlook, or culture.

Some employees prefer looking at the big picture; others thrive by focusing on small details. Certain employees are more people-oriented, whereas their counterparts would rather concentrate on tasks. Some people relish the limelight, but others find satisfaction working behind the scenes.

Health care management has long rejected diverse viewpoints, considering them as threats to the status quo. The managers' intentions were often admirable. In their minds, standardization was needed to ensure safety. However, standardization has failed in all spheres. We have lost the innovation that we needed to remain financially solvent and have not even improved safety, with our medical error rate at an all-time high.

Excessive paperwork was generated during the 1980s and 1990s in an attempt to standardize care and improve safety. However, this merely served to consume a lot of time and took nurses away from providing safe care to their patients.

Diversity builds profitability. Organizations have lost valuable market data that could have prevented our current financial problems. When managers cut costs without listening to nurses, they sowed the seeds of our current nursing crisis. Nurses haven't volunteered to offer suggestions and innovative ideas because they have been censured so many times for having a different perspective. So now, in many facilities, nurses rarely even report many of their concerns.

Organizations must satisfy customer needs if they want to remain competitive. But before satisfying those needs, managers must know what those needs are. Managers of organizations need to listen to frontline nurses—the ones who listen to patients the most. This will enable managers of organizations to create the kinds of services that consumers want. Having continual streams of ideas from frontline employees such as nurses ensures financial viability and keeps you ahead of the competition.

Diversity also reduces risk. A balanced mix of personalities decreases risk because everyone looks at various aspects of each problem differently. For example, a seminar participant recounted some workplace conflicts resulting from her manager's habit of focusing on the big picture, whereas she liked centering on the details. When encouraged to think back to situations when her focus on detail paid off, her face suddenly lit up. "Yes, my organization was sued several years ago, and it was my detailed written notes that provided the necessary documentation needed to win the case." In this instance, both the manager and employee were able to reduce their risk because of their diversity of temperaments.

Respect for diversity is the foundation of innovation, yet the health care environment has not been very kind to innovators. The powerful status quo usually squashes many novel ideas. You can counteract this tendency by providing a nurturing environment so that innovators can survive. Innovation represents the bridge to our future. Good managers encourage collaboration between innovators and less inventive employees. Each learns from the other so that both can become more successful.

Diversity is also necessary for teamwork. Teams that represent all personality styles perform better. Their different perspectives help teams overcome obstacles and add value to their organization.

Showcase your diversity. Suppose you have a nurse who excels at categorizing things. With good humor, recognize her by saying,

"Cindy color-coded all of our keys to save us all a little bit of valuable time." And remember to say thank you. Everyone on your staff needs sincere appreciation.

Five Ways to Capitalize on Diversity by Focusing Inward

1. Assess your own self-esteem. Low self-esteem is a lens that distorts the actions of others. Staff with low self-esteem are likely to assess people incorrectly and undermine them. Some people think that if the other person is right, then they must be wrong. A struggle about who is right and who is wrong ensues in order to protect the person's fragile self-esteem. This kind of competition and sabotage occurs frequently in health care. Skilled nurse managers can end it by making sure that everyone has an equal chance to participate.

2. Examine your attitude. People fear change and spend an enormous amount of energy fighting it. Because corporate structures change frequently, ask yourself, "Is this change an innovative way to improve services or is it a threat to basic values such as honesty and commitment to quality?" In the first case, go with the flow. But oppose the change in the second case.

3. Change yourself first. We influence others more than we think. An authoritarian approach creates dependency. On the other hand, a staff-friendly culture cultivates the independence that is necessary for staff to use all of their abilities.

4. Be flexible. Good policies create quality and consistency. But policies are written in black and white, whereas human situations come in shades of gray. Use critical thinking if a policy doesn't make sense. Policies should serve the customer, not the other way around. Organizations should hire professionals to use their judgment and interpret policies on an individual basis.

5. Have a sense of humor. Humor decreases stress and improves teamwork. Friendly teasing about differences can actually bond staff members to each other. "That's a good job for you, Sara. I know you'll take care of every detail."

Five Ways to Capitalize on Diversity by Focusing Outward

1. Understand diversity. We tend to compare ourselves with others. If others are different, some people automatically think they

are wrong. A better approach is to reframe the situation and ask yourself, "What can I learn from this person?"

2. Show respect. Respect empowers people because it allows them to be authentic. Staff are more innovative and productive when they can be themselves.

3. Communicate effectively. People with different personalities need different approaches. Choose one that matches the other person's expectations. In other words, don't be a one-trick pony. Learn various communication styles so that you can pick the best one for each situation. If you have one or two styles, you may be effective in 25% to 35% of situations. If you have six to eight styles, you have a good chance of being effective in every situation.

4. Seek areas of agreement. Search for ways to agree. A list of agreements makes it easier to create enough momentum to overcome points of disagreement. Focusing on the positive can actually make it happen.

5. Collaborate. Collaboration is more successful in a diverse environment because of the multitude of ideas from which to choose. When people say, "These results are better than any member of the team could have produced alone," you know that you have achieved success.

I attended my clinical nursing education in New York City at a hospital with a substantial Hispanic population. We learned to speak Spanish, and we were taught how to be the right kind of nurse for our patients.

One lesson that I learned was to be flexible. We were asked to listen well, to look at each situation individually, and to remain sensitive to cultural differences. For example, our Hispanic patients were accustomed to maternity practices that, at first, seemed foreign to us. But we didn't try to impose our own ideas on them. As we examined their customs, we discovered that most of their customs were just different ways to accomplish the same goals that were in our texts. Occasionally, we made some suggestions to improve the care of their infants. But mostly, we genuinely respected them, built warm relationships, and shared in the joy that they experienced with the birth of their children.

Assess how you can make better use of the diverse ideas of your staff. Look inward and outward for ways to promote diversity. Welcome people with different personalities and beliefs so that you and your organization can benefit from the magic of the staffing mix.

Promoting Diversity

TIPS FOR CLINICAL NURSES

- Avoid feeling threatened by diversity.
- Be flexible.
- Understand others.
- Seek agreement.
- Avoid defensiveness.

TIPS FOR MANAGERS

- Question standardized protocols, in order to reduce waste.
- Share power.
- Be adaptable.
- Showcase diversity.
- Use diversity to decrease risk.

TIPS FOR EDUCATORS

- Accept diverse points of view.
- Use experiential strategies.
- Decrease standardization for students.
- Stimulate multiple solutions to challenges.
- Encourage students to speak up.

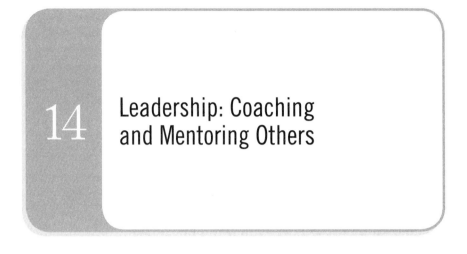

14 Leadership: Coaching and Mentoring Others

We can't solve problems by using the same kind of thinking we used when we created them. —*Albert Einstein*

The health care industry has the talent but lacks the vision to make the leap that Einstein suggests. Caregivers would like to provide safe and thorough care, but they have been unable to overcome systems problems that have blocked individual effort. Our health care system has not only failed patients; it has also failed nurses, who try every day to provide safe, caring, and cost-effective patient care.

We need leaders with the vision to show us the way to health care excellence. Smart Nursing core values—respect, integrity, flexibility, simplicity, professional culture, communication, and caring—are the stepping stones to excellence.

- Imagine leaders who can transcend our differences and bring a sense of calm to a chaotic world.
- Imagine leaders who understand that patient-care excellence depends on the commitment of frontline staff.
- Imagine leaders who are able to build a health care community powered by the renewal of the hearts and minds of the staff.

Daniel Goleman sums it up well in his book *Primal Leadership*: "People need to see, feel, and touch the values and vision of the organization . . . [They] need to feel as if they can reach for the organization's dream without compromising their own" (Goleman, 2002).

Practicing Smart Nursing core values determines, to a large extent, a leader's credibility. The acid test of credibility is whether the staff even pay attention to what their leaders say. I have seen employee groups numbering in the hundreds, who were dutifully present at hour-long presentations by senior managers yet not believing even one word because leadership actions rarely matched the words. What they see from their leaders does not match what they hear.

Can You Be a Leader if You Are Not a Manager?

Think of the most competent managers you have known. Were they successful because of their position or because of their expertise and humanity? Although managers use positional power, such as in the hiring process, the best managers depend on a stronger kind of power—"expert power"—to influence their staff. People with a wealth of knowledge have expert power because others naturally respect them and want to learn from them. Suppose that a manager wants a staff member to take a certain action. Using positional power would compel an employee to respond, but expert power would persuade the employee to respond, which is a stronger result, because the employee would want to take the action.

Clinical nurses can access the same expert power as managers because they, too, have expertise. Expert power has the added advantage of growing every time that you learn something new.

Shared Governance

Shared governance, project management, and interdepartmental collaboration are only three of the leadership opportunities that are available to nonmanagers. For instance, a knowledgeable clinical nurse with good people-skills might be given decision-making staffing authority as part of a shared governance initiative. Another nurse might be asked to head up a patient safety project. Clinical nurses might also lead their departments to forge better relationships with physicians or other departments.

An example of an expert clinical nurse with decision-making authority is a charge nurse who can add or subtract a staff member without having his or her decision approved. Expert nurses have the judgment to make smart staffing decisions

An example of leadership at the bedside is when expert nurses make decisions at the point of care during a clinical emergency. The nurse makes his or her expectation clear that the physician will respond to this reasoned assessment in a timely way.

Leading Staff in a Culture of Safety

Creating a culture of safety requires a partnership between leaders and staff. Amy Vogelsmeier, a geriatric nursing scholar at the University of Missouri, describes the shared values and outcomes of this partnership:

> "Nurse leaders should liberate staff to do the right thing, using their own skills and talents. Health care organizations should leverage their workforce so that many eyes are searching for errors" (Vogelsmeier, 2007).

Many eyes should be searching for errors, and, because clinical nurses are the ones that see so much, their leadership is important. If you ask yourself, "Who am I to be a leader?" listen to what Gerry Spence says about credibility:

> Question: No one listens to me, Why should they? Who am I?
> Answer: Anyone can be credible, but we must risk telling the truth— about ourselves.
> To win, we must be believed.
> To be believed, we must be believable.
> To be believable, we must tell the truth.
> That is where we must focus, in that rare, rich place, that nucleus of our being. That is the magical place where credibility dwells. (Spence, 1995)

The National Patient Safety Foundation recommends that clinical nurses participate in leadership: "Nurses must be actively engaged as leaders in the development and implementation of changes and improvements in health care safety."

How Does the Leader of a Band of Caring Staff Find Wisdom?

Capable leaders exhibit candor, humor, and a sincere respect for differences. Emotional and social intelligence add to the empathy and confidence that radiate from them.

After contemplating the sheer magnitude of his responsibilities, one supervisor commented, "I have to know how to do many things, or I have to know many people who know how to do many things." Every day, this successful supervisor recognizes that building relationships enables him to draw from an endless stream of talent. He respects the clinical expertise of his staff, empowering them to make independent decisions within their scope of practice.

One way that supervisors tap the knowledge of expert clinical nurses is during a crisis regarding the need to float staff. Many times, clinical nurses are the ones who come up with the most common sense solutions.

Effective leaders ensure that each department of their organization is aligned with the others. What matters most is that organizational goals are not just put in a policy manual but also put into practice. Conflict between departments is a common health care problem that is caused by a lack of alignment. Although frontline staff can facilitate collaboration by the way that they treat people in other departments, it is the responsibility of leaders above the departmental level to recognize harmful conflict and to take appropriate action.

Nursing outcomes have become more important than ever to the entire organization.

> Magnet Force 1 recommends that nursing leaders, at all levels of the organization, convey a strong sense of advocacy and support for the staff and for the patients (ANCC).

Pay for Performance

In October 2008, The Center for Medicare and Medicaid Services (CMS) will stop reimbursing hospitals for eight hospital-acquired conditions. This concept of "pay for performance" is described on the NQF Web site (www.qualityforum.org). It explains that payment is used as a mechanism to incentivize or reward higher quality of care—so-called pay for performance programs—and to determine what design strategies or other characteristics of these programs are known to produce the desired outcome. In other words, CMS wants to discover the best practices and then reward those that use them.

Four of the pay for performance identifiers are related to nursing care—pressure ulcers, patient falls, urinary tract infections, and vascular access infections—thus making nursing outcomes more important than ever. Medicare will use these identifiers to determine payment as will many insurance companies.

Wise Decisions at the Point of Care

An autonomous nurse at a patient's bedside exemplifies the principle of Magnet Force 9: the nurse is expected to practice autonomously, as is consistent with professional standards.

One of a leader's most important roles is to help frontline employees excel. When employees are enthusiastic and energetic, their talents bubble up at the point of care. To achieve this goal, health care managers must delegate enough authority so that clinical staff are able to respond quickly to patient needs. The second step of delegation is to follow up to make sure that the nurse understands the project and is making good progress.

Delegation prepares nurses to become future leaders. As nurses operate with greater authority, they experience professional growth and gain new skills so that they can teach others and benefit their entire organization.

When managers delegate wisely, they can significantly reduce their own workloads. Instead of managing crises, their time—spent on building relationships and addressing the root causes of problems—helps every clinical nurse on the staff because problems don't consistently recur. Managers who delegate decision-making authority also find that staffing issues take less time, because the staff works hard to make the schedule function well. Empowered clinical nurses enjoy higher job satisfaction; control of their own work environment enables them to solve problems without going up and down a long chain of command. Patients are more satisfied as well because their needs are promptly met and with greater regard for their individuality.

> Daniel Goleman supports this approach with the following advice: "Institutions that endure thrive not because of one leader's charisma, but because they cultivate leadership throughout the system" (Goleman, 2002).

Do More with Less

Promoting individual freedom and avoiding micromanagement release energy that can be channeled into constructive actions. As with other tools, we need to use this process wisely. The art of knowing how much structure to retain is important for managers at every level. As the management span of control (the number of people that a manager supervises) becomes flatter, there are often only four levels in the administrative hierarchy: frontline employee (nurse), frontline manager (nurse manager), department head (vice president of nursing), and senior manager (CEO).

Leading a lean organization, in which employees are empowered to transform waste into constructive improvements, is also an art because lean is not the same as chronically understaffed. A key difference between the two is that staff satisfaction is high in lean organizations because there is enough staff to provide quality care. Lean organizations generate a sense of staff pride and the joy of seeing one's innovations comes to fruition. Employees in lean organizations enjoy a vitalizing cycle of energy and enthusiasm. However, chronically understaffed facilities exhaust their staff, mentally and physically, and find that their staff members experience a vicious cycle, one that results in nurse burnout and turnover.

The AHRQ describes "lean" this way, "Although the term *lean* suggests that the core focus of this approach is increased efficiency, the true focus of lean is on evolving to a state in which work processes relentlessly emphasize eliminating waste. Waste is defined as acts that do not add value to customers and includes wasted resources, time, and human spirit" (Hughes, 2008).

Managers also retain responsibility for the end result when they delegate decision-making authority to clinical nurses. Several guidelines to follow include:

- Give your staff enough time and staffing assistance when delegating authority.
- Coach your staff so that they have the skills needed for effectiveness. (See the coaching ideas at the end of this chapter.)
- Teach your staff to look at the big picture so that their efforts are aligned with those of senior management.
- Work with new nurses until they have the skills to accept delegation. (See Chapter 17, "Becoming a Lifelong Learner: How to Accelerate Your Professional Development.")
- Support your nurses and periodically plan informal conversations to develop the decision-making skills of clinical nurses.
- Build solid relationships with your staff and with those in other departments.

Relationships shape the foundation of leadership, and trust binds the components of this foundation together. This process builds a sense of community that enables nurses to function at their full professional capacity.

The Gallup organization found that no single factor more clearly predicts the productivity of an employee than his relationship with his direct supervisor. (Loehr, 2003)

Trust

Gallup's data on the employee-supervisor relationship say that this relationship depends on trust, because trust is a common denominator of successful leadership. Trust energizes employees and speeds up work processes, enabling smart leaders to unleash employee potential.
Harkins (1999) describes

trust as "the currency of leadership"—an asset with an unlimited return.

Trust is not seen as merely the byproduct of relationships. It is viewed as the "goal of a leader's relationships" (quoted in Morath, 2004). When staff members trust their leaders, they don't have to waste time and energy judging complex political implications every time that their leader makes a decision.

Less successful leaders fail to recognize such opportunities. Those who insist on overseeing everything themselves have little time left for their most important work and are unavailable when the staff really need their help. Besides wasting time and money, this kind of micromanagement sends a negative message of distrust.

Suppose that Joe, a supervisor, gives Sally a specific responsibility. If Sally's coworkers, Suzie, Sam, and Marsha, don't trust Joe, they would probably have a discussion about whether Joe might be playing favorites and the staff would waste precious time and energy looking for hidden agendas. Employees have sensitive antennae about leader credibility and often spend inordinate amounts of time filling in information for the grapevine. I have seen employees dutifully attend important meetings but not believe a single word of what their leaders said. But if employees know from experience that Joe is trustworthy and fair, they can take his requests at face value and act on them. It's no wonder that trust multiplies productivity.

Managing employee energy is a concept that is not always discussed but one that is directly related to employee productivity and health care costs. Jim Loehr, in his book *The Power of Full Engagement*, explains the relationship of employee energy and leadership:

> "Great leaders are stewards of organizational energy . . . they must mobilize, focus, invest, channel, renew, and expand the energy of others" (Loehr, 2003).

Following their company's vision and mission statements is the common drive that employees follow. Extraordinary organizations have ethical leaders, who use the core values of Smart Nursing to build credibility, thus motivating others to jump onboard. System changes often start with a groundswell and build up to a tipping point, when those who were reluctant at first are willing to step onboard. As we welcome employees whose thoughts percolate up from the frontline, we can only imagine how many multiple solutions will evolve.

Look at the system dynamics:

> A complex adaptive system is a collection of individuals who have the freedom to act . . . Orderly behavior can emerge among many agents who are acting independently but who share a common drive. (Palmer et al., 2003)

The best leaders share power and build work improvement by coaching and mentoring their employees. They replicate their passion for leadership by encouraging each staff member to seek his or her own individual style.

Five Ways to Use Coaching and Mentoring to Retain Employees

1. Use "stay interviews." Some companies enjoy high retention because managers take time to talk with employees about remaining onboard. One employee who experienced a stay interview described it this way: "It makes a difference to have something other than your standard review. And, I feel appreciated when my manager takes the extra time."
2. Ask yourself the following question: "Are my employees receiving a good return on their investment of time, talent, and money?" When 25 global talent leaders got together for a think tank, key issues regarding employee engagement and retention were discussed. One of their key findings was that employees need to

feel that they have a return on their investment in the company (Kaye, 2003).

3. Give your nurses enough support. Many nurses think of safer ways to perform their job, but they won't contribute those ideas without support. Mentors are in a good position to promote staff safety initiatives.

4. Identify employee dissatisfaction early. Mentors are in an ideal position to monitor staff satisfaction. They notice the beginning of staff cynicism early. When mentors are unable to intervene, they know how to find someone else who can respond to the situation.

5. Be a good role model. The CEOs and the nursing directors should be the finest mentoring models. Employees respond well to seeing clear corporate values in action and having a model of excellence to live up to.

One excellent nurse leader was in the process of handling a common clinical situation that led to a discussion to understand better the details of the situation. I made the following observations: The leader avoided a confrontational approach and kept an open mind, to absorb accurately the details of the situation. But she did not gloss over potential sources of conflict. Instead, she used systematic open- and close-ended questions to obtain an abundance of accurate information. Her attitude also reduced defensiveness and facilitated employee growth. This leader later shared her thoughts with me.

I am always one who wants the truth and who respects the truth from my staff. We can learn more about what happened than what was reported to us. Sometimes these things take on a life of their own. I am a firm believer that everyone should learn problem-solving and decision-making skills. My job is so much more than being a manager. It is being a leader and a role model. Staff who work in this type of environment can perform at their full professional capacity.

Strategic plans are more meaningful when you involve clinical nurses using the following techniques:

1. Hold focus groups, composed of nurses, to elucidate valuable nursing perspectives.

2. Ask for positive and negative feedback regarding your organizational culture and how it affects nurse productivity.

3. Review your corporate values. Do you practice these values consistently? Are they compatible with staff values? If not, why not?

4. Invite your clinical nurses to share their ideas on nurse recruitment and retention and on other important issues.

5. Discuss the benefits for all staff members when nurses share their skills with each other.

6. Ask yourself, "Do I identify my nurses' skills in my strategic plan?" You should know what skills your nurses have. (See the skill assessment sheet in the appendix.)

   ■ Which nurses are cross-trained?

   ■ What nonclinical skills, computer literacy, artistic ability, or public speaking are available to you?

   ■ How can you best support information sharing? Reward nurses who are willing to utilize a large number of their skills. When nurses are generous with their abilities, managers should be generous in return.

   ■ Align nursing with other departments.

   ■ Successful organizations know how to induce staff in their departments to work together. They use synergy to raise productivity. This means that no department is more important than another and that they therefore avoid turf wars.

   ■ What attracts and retains exceptional talent?

   ■ The best nurses want to work with competent peers who are similarly interested in excellence. Many times, these exceptional nurses recruit others like themselves because they value working in such positive environments.

   ■ Expand your employees' capabilities.

   ■ What are the effective rewards for lifelong learners? If you are a clinical nurse, become a lifelong learner so that you have more to offer your employer.

   ■ Cultivate new leaders. Teach the components of leadership—communication, respect, and vision. Let your staff practice on small projects and give them feedback.

BEST PRACTICE: SUCCESSFUL COACHING IN ACTION

Linda Pullins, VP, Marion General Hospital, Marion, OH

At Marion General Hospital, in Marion, Ohio, great changes are evident, as the result of two years of intense work with the nursing staff. Morale was at an all-time low: there were unfilled nurse manager positions, near-misses were rising, and agency staffing costs were through the roof, with so many unfilled RN positions.

Linda Pullins, Vice President of Patient-Care Services, planned a bold move that would take some of her best nurses out of bedside staffing and other positions into the role of professional coaches, in an effort to get to the root problem of what was going on in patient care. Nurses were invited to participate in a one-year initiative that would place them directly at the bedside, working with RNs to improve their care management and critical-thinking skills. All were guaranteed that they could transfer back into their original positions at the end of one year.

A proposal was shared with the CEO and Medical Staff Executive Committee that would entail hiring additional agency nurse staffing to cover some of the positions. Outcomes and success measures were identified, along with metrics to measure along the way. The idea of pulling good nurses away from taking care of patients was met with resistance and disdain at various levels. The idea of bringing in some select consultant interventions also was met with skepticism. Why couldn't we just fix this ourselves?

Linda knew that this was not going to be a quick fix; patient care had not gotten to this level overnight, and she needed to be clear on the priorities for the coaches. The professional coaches spent three weeks in didactic and classroom discussions, learning about emotional intelligence, how coaching was different from precepting, how we would address the numerous problems that they would encounter, and how the staff would accept them.

Within six months, the start of a turnaround was apparent; the coaches would share their own stories and examples of how far both they and the staff had come. This was certainly not an easy journey, nor was every week filled with successes. Many tears were shed, along with many good laughs, but the joy of taking care of patients was coming back to Marion General!

Marion General now enjoys the following: Press Ganey Patient Satisfaction has moved from the 4th to the 86th percentile on the inpatient survey. Retention is now at 94%. Employer of Choice scores from the employees is at a five-year high, and 56 RNs were successfully recruited in one year—three times the normal recruitment! Our patients, staff, physicians, and new employees tell us that there is something different about Marion General.

It can happen, but it must happen at the bedside, with nurses and managers working side by side to deal with the stressful and complicated care issues of today. We are a better organization, and we are taking better care of our patients with this work. As Arthur Ashe once said, "To achieve greatness, start where you are. Use what you have. Do what you can."

Promoting Leadership

TIPS FOR CLINICAL NURSES

- Build leadership skills.
- View leadership as a challenge.
- Follow up on your initiatives.
- Seek accountability.
- Be generous with praise and support.

TIPS FOR MANAGERS

- Use relationships to connect with your staff.
- Build consensus.
- Create a shared vision.
- Value your intellectual capital.
- Use nurses to increase your organization's success.

TIPS FOR EDUCATORS

- Be a leadership role model.
- Maintain frequent contact with nurse leaders.
- Give students feedback on their leadership work.
- Encourage students to follow current health care leadership issues.
- Encourage students to build a vision for the future.

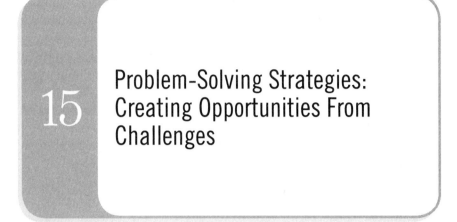

15

Problem-Solving Strategies: Creating Opportunities From Challenges

Your world will be different, and I can't teach you how to solve the problems you will encounter. But I can teach you how to think. If you know how to think, you can solve any problem that comes your way.
—Fritz Bendel, 1955 (Author's Father)

Within every problem lie the seeds of opportunity. Our many health care challenges constitute important opportunities for all health care professionals. Sowing seeds of opportunity is important, but the course of change is not always even. Innovation often follows a failure. The seeds need time to take root and grow. Clinical staff members are well positioned to develop solutions because they see the problems firsthand, and health care executives without clinical experiences need the perspectives of clinical staff to be effective leaders.

This chapter describes the process of transforming problems into opportunities by examining basic problem-solving strategies and then suggesting how those strategies can be applied to health care. The quantum approach to problem solving is considered, as well as the linear approach. Most specific suggestions have elements of both approaches.

Using your thoughts to solve basic linear problems involves analysis and synthesis. Analysis occurs when you break a complex whole down into simpler elements. Synthesis is the reverse, a process of recombining basic elements to form the same outcome—or to form another complex outcome.

Think about the following simple analogy of analysis using ordinary saline. When you break saline down partially, into its elements, you get salt and water. To break it down completely, into its most elemental form, you must also break the water down into hydrogen and oxygen and the salt into sodium and chlorine.

A health care example of using a linear and nonlinear comparison is the examination of relationships. Relationships are complex processes involving trust, respect, and other components. Each of those components can be broken down further. For example, respect can be broken down into self-love, open-mindedness, and other qualities.

Synthesis is the process of recombining the basic elements. In the case of saline, you can recombine the salt and water to get saline again, you can recombine them differently to get stronger saline or a less concentrated version, or you can add other substances such as sugar and get dextrose with saline.

In the case of relationships, trust and respect can be combined to form good relationships or you can add improved communication techniques to form even stronger and better relationships. But because trust, relationships, and communication result from complex adaptive systems as well, they have many nonlinear qualities.

Many of the concepts in Smart Nursing are the result of breaking down issues into simpler forms and then exchanging those ideas between different disciplines, such as education and business. This is a linear approach, but since these issues are part of complex adaptive systems, a linear approach is not enough; quantum and systemic approaches are required in order to understand them. The use of bar codes to improve patient safety is an example of a practice from another discipline being successfully adopted by health care.

A book describing the unity of knowledge on a larger scale is *Consilience: The Unity of Knowledge* by Pulitzer Prize-winning author Edward O. Wilson. Wilson shows that natural sciences, social sciences, and mathematics have common components. The purchase of an ordinary Megabucks lottery ticket is an example of consilience. When you decide to buy a ticket, you use both mathematics and psychology. Your choice involves assessing the probability of winning (mathematics) and your attitude toward risk (psychology). For example, are you a risk taker or a risk-averse person?

Health Care Challenges

You can use this process to transform health care challenges into opportunities by creating your own innovations. Review some of the following health care challenges: safety, role change, productivity, and innovation. These challenges are the source of many nursing opportunities.

Safety

Nurses are risk managers. They notice potential problems early and build positive patient relationships. Solving problems early allows organizations to decrease their risk, because early nursing interventions prevent patient injury. In the event that an error does occur, patients who have developed good relationships with staff are less likely to sue. Patients often start litigation because they feel that "no one cared."

Organizations have caused many of their own safety problems by using heavy-handed tactics to increase nurse productivity. One of these tactics is the "speed-up." Speed-ups require nurses to work faster without regard for consequences. Speed-ups have become an obstacle to patient safety, because they have caused nurse fatigue and prevented nurses from assessing patients often enough. Smart Nursing strategies remove this kind of obstacle to productivity and allow nurses to work smarter instead of just faster. This is one reason why Smart Nursing strategies are more important than ever.

- Quantify the role of nursing as frontline risk managers. A nurse who prevents litigation may save the organization more than $500,000.
- Empower nurses to make safety decisions at the patient level.
- Provide safe staffing levels.

If you are a nurse manager or charge nurse, you have many opportunities to improve safety.

- Express your perspective to senior management.
- Support your nurses, prevent burnout, and show your organization how you can increase productivity with autonomous nurses.

Role Change

Times are changing. In the future, nursing roles will become more advisory and less regulatory. The Internet has enabled patients to collect abundant data but does not help them acquire the skills needed to interpret this proliferation of information. Patients need professional advice to enable them to make smart health care decisions. Nurses are ideally positioned to be advisors to patients and to advise their own leaders.

NURSES ARE BEST POSITIONED TO FILL EMERGING ADVISORY ROLES

To fulfill these roles, nurses need to expand their outlook. They need to envision management's big picture, as well as their own perspectives, and to think about the larger context affecting these issues. Many times, nurses with legitimate requests limit their success by viewing issues only from their own individual perspective.

Nurses know that patient-care success depends on framing their explanations in terms of the patient's point of view. The same is true with management.

Nursing is an important part of your organization's investment in human resources. In the past, facilities have slashed nursing budgets unreasonably. Cost cutting may be necessary, but nurses can best advise their organizations about where to make the cuts without reducing the quality of care. Nurses may advise management to forego expensive building or redecoration in favor of scheduling an adequate number of clinical staff. Listen to them. Act on their reasoned recommendations

Nursing, the most respected of all professions, builds patient trust. Nurses notice patient needs because they spend the most time listening to patients. At present, we are losing this important patient information. Organizations need to capture this data because it is valuable market research. Nurses who advise their organizations are able to identify new services that are needed by patients. For example, nurses and social workers first identified the need for subacute units as described in Chapter 8, "Communication."

When patients complain about gaps in medical services, explore those complaints. Consider them as important pieces of market research. Then, reframe those complaints into opportunities. Suppose that the patients complain about lack of transportation. Bring those complaints to management and reframe them into opportunities. For instance, this may be a good opportunity to start a new shuttle service or to add stops to an existing one.

Frame your requests in terms of benefits to your organization and show that your requests bring value. For example,

"My request will attract new patients."

"Although this idea will cost $1,000 to implement, it will decrease expenses by $2,200 annually."

"If you change from X to Y, you will double the return on your investment."

Productivity

Productivity is one of our most important issues. Management has tried to raise productivity the wrong way—by insisting that nurses care for too many patients. This practice has caused a rapid rise in our medical error rate and decreased nurse productivity; overworked nurses complete less work, not more.

However, the pressure for high nurse productivity will continue because of escalating medical costs. What we need is more collaboration between nurses and managers to find ways to improve nurse productivity without raising the medical error rate. Nurses, as frontline employees, notice ways to streamline their practice in their day-to-day work. Sometimes these potential improvements seem too small to bother with and the nursing staff disregards them. But minor changes are important. For example, when nurses share small improvements, the discussion often stimulates other nurses to add their ideas. Before you know it, they come up with faster ways to work.

Suppose that you find a way to save 10 minutes. When you multiply the 10 minutes by only 100 nurses and then by 365 days, you end up with over 6,000 hours saved per year. From my experience, the best organizations have employees who create continuous streams of small innovations.

If more nurses adopted this philosophy and were supported by their employers, patients would be able to receive safe care without as much cost.

Innovation

Every nurse can innovate. Assess your own strengths and weaknesses and then choose to participate in the opportunities that spark your interest.

People gravitate toward certain areas, melding their experiences with their own interests. Be open to new experiences. Be willing to accept opportunities by turning weaknesses into strengths.

In 1995, health care problems resulted in my own reconsideration of nursing as a career. But I reframed the problem into an opportunity. I thought to myself, "Health care problems could be an opportunity for nurses who are willing to work toward positive change." I knew that, in order to be successful, I needed better skills of influence.

If you feel limited regarding skills of influence, master them. These are learnable skills. I learned public speaking by joining Toastmasters. You can do it too. I learned to write for publication by joining a local writers group. You can do the same. Use the nursing shortage as motivation to learn new skills and to change your work environment.

> Health care problems are an opportunity for nurses who are willing to work toward positive change.

Ask yourself what issues are most important.

- Do you want to focus on building a more respectful workplace?
- Do you want to lobby for more autonomy?
- Do you want to participate in marketing?

Identify the skills that you need to learn. Make a plan, take action, and then go ahead and learn them. No time? I learned these skills while I was working 44 hours a week as a nurse, taking call one day a week, driving two teenage children to all of their activities, and going to graduate school one night a week for five years.

I devised the "hour-a-day plan," spending one hour a day on my project six days a week. I did my homework when my daughters were doing theirs. Try it. You will be amazed at what you will be able to accomplish.

If you are willing to accept these opportunities, you might need to examine the way that you learn. Knowing their own learning style helps people to become more successful students.

Focus on the following actions to maximize your personal and professional growth:

- Nurture your natural curiosity.
- Become a lifelong learner.
- Be persistent.

Nurture Your Natural Curiosity

We are all naturally curious as children. As we mature, we tend to lose this childlike curiosity to varying degrees. Nurturing your natural curiosity reconnects you to your creativity and provides you with new opportunities. Your patient safety record will probably improve when you exercise your natural curiosity, because it prompts you to follow up on your hunches. Have you ever noticed something odd about a patient? Has natural curiosity led you to check out those symptoms? Haven't you averted medical errors when your curiosity compelled you to check things out? Using your natural curiosity also keeps you young at heart. A curious mind rejuvenates people, keeps them young, and promotes healthy living.

One way to start restoring your professional curiosity is by brainstorming, which can be done individually as well as in groups.

- Choose a topic that interests you.
- Choose a day when you have a few hours of free time.
- Find a quiet spot.
- Clear your mind, and open it to new ideas.
- Write down all of your ideas without judging them—you can weed out the impractical ones later.

Suppose that you witness an incident of disrespect and want to take action. Start brainstorming and see how many action ideas you can generate. I came up with the following 13 ideas in just three minutes. You could probably generate many more ideas if you take more time. Write down every idea. Here are some sample actions to respond to disrespectful behavior:

1. Build staff self-esteem.
2. Use humor.
3. Be assertive.
4. Talk with the offender privately.
5. Talk with the nurse manger.
6. Talk with senior management.
7. Ask senior management to come to the unit and witness the offensive behavior.
8. Write an article about respect in your newsletter.
9. Recommend that the education department offer classes on anger management.

10. Work with other departments and take group action.
11. Address this issue at a meeting of your professional association.
12. Collaborate with physicians.
13. File a complaint with the offender's licensure board.

Now, give brainstorming a try yourself. Clear your mind and then take 5 or 10 minutes to brainstorm about one of the following topics, or choose another topic:

- Increasing nurse productivity
- Working with management as partners
- Using nurses as risk managers
- Recognizing nurses as marketers

Take out a sheet of paper and number the lines from 1 to 25. Write your topic on the top and start brainstorming, writing down all of your ideas. Then prioritize your ideas by numbering them 1 through 25 according to how much they interest you. Review the top 5 and consider how much each topic is needed by your organization or by the health care industry in general. Then choose one or two ideas to pursue further and take action.

Become a Lifelong Learner

Nurses need to keep learning throughout their lives. Articles in every industry worldwide recommend that employees be lifelong learners. It is the best way to manage change and to remain employable. Nurses who have failed to expand their skills have contributed to the nursing crisis. Health care is a rapidly changing industry. Nurses need to keep up clinically, but they also need to become just as proficient with skills of influence—such as communication, negotiation, and persuasion.

Be willing to step outside your comfort zone. Too often, people feel reluctant to try new skills because they enjoy a feeling of security within familiar environments. So they wait to change until they have to. They consider their comfort zones as secure sanctuaries and limit their chances for success. Learning new skills provides intellectual stimulation. People need intellectual stimulation to thrive, not just to survive. As a result, lifelong learners tend to be among the happy people; they continue their journey of personal and professional growth throughout their lives.

Be Persistent

When you learn a new skill, it is easy to get discouraged. Everyone experiences doubts when others exceed their skill level. It is all right to take "baby steps." The secrets to succeeding with learning new information are to be persistent, use positive self-talk, and reward yourself every now and then.

The process of learning something new can be slow in the beginning until you reach a critical mass. You must put forth a large effort for a small reward; after you reach the critical mass, you will achieve larger rewards with smaller efforts. Eventually, you will have learned enough to start feeling competent. You will need more practice to achieve excellence, but you are on your way at that point.

Use positive self-talk along the way, such as the following: "Of course, I still make some mistakes. I am a beginner at this. No one was born with this skill. Everyone was a beginner at one time, just like me. Eventually, I will be an expert in this skill."

Give yourself a reward after you have succeeded with one of your baby steps. Take an afternoon off, get a manicure, and plan lunch with a friend. Rewards help you enjoy the process and celebrate each level of your success.

Remember, opportunity knocks, and it is knocking loudly on nursing's door. But nothing will happen until you take action. You must open the door to opportunity if you would like to enjoy this kind of success.

Turning Problems Into Opportunities

TIPS FOR CLINICAL NURSES

- Be creative.
- Rethink common practices.
- Look for an easy way, without sacrificing safety or quality.
- Read widely.
- Question the status quo.

TIPS FOR MANAGERS

- Use group brainstorming.
- Maintain strong connections with senior management and communicate nursing input.
- Increase the return on your human resource investment.

- Support staff problem solving.
- Encourage group projects to take advantage of synergy.

TIPS FOR EDUCATORS

- Teach analysis, synthesis, and quantum approaches to issues.
- Look for input from other industries.
- Value multiple solutions to problems.
- Focus on future needs.
- Prioritize health care challenges.

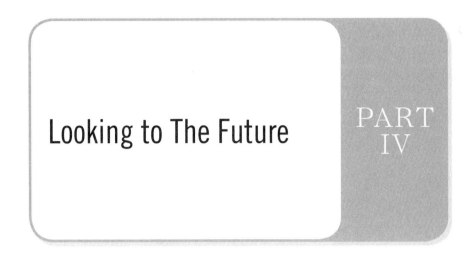

Looking to The Future

PART
IV

16	**Benefits to Groups Outside Nursing: How CEOs, Physicians, Trustees, and Managed Care Professionals Can Help**

Seek first to understand, then to be understood.   *—Stephen R. Covey*

Why Non-Nurses Should Be Interested in Smart Nursing

Health care needs many perspectives to solve the nursing crisis. Consumers, physicians, CEOs, and trustees are more effective if they have a good understanding of nursing issues. This understanding promotes better management and more effective interactions with nurses.

The stakes are high: Health care costs are increasing, and the medical error rate has escalated. Many nurses have left health care, and physicians are also being squeezed by the system. The CEOs and the trustees have the frustrating task of retaining nursing staff while trying to balance their budgets. These problems are especially difficult in health care.

Consider some of Smart Nursing's benefits to various non-nurse groups:

Benefits to Consumers

- Patients receive safer care with high RN-to-patient ratios. Research described in the introduction to this book confirms that even one additional patient added to an RN's assignment substantially raises the complication rate for both medical and surgical patients.

- Satisfaction levels climb when patients receive timely nursing interventions.
- Education provided by nurses promotes wellness.
- Simplified procedures are easy for patients to understand.
- Flexibility enables patients to receive care that is designed for their individual needs.

Benefits to Physicians

- Physicians improve their own quality of care when alert nurses report potential complications that enable physicians to intervene quickly.
- Nursing perspectives added to medical viewpoints promote comprehensive patient care.
- Nurse-physician partnerships save time, as when nurses quickly summarize patient events for physicians.
- With enough nurses, physicians can expand their medical practices to meet patient need.
- Physician delegation to nurses reduces medical cost.

Benefits to CEOs and Trustees

- Nurses are the most trusted professionals within your organization. They build positive relationships with your customers.
- Nurses are your organization's frontline risk managers. They notice potential problems early enough to prevent injury. Listen to them.
- Excellent patient care and high patient satisfaction attract new patients.
- High staff satisfaction reduces human resource outlays.
- Nurses are valuable market researchers. Patient requests often indicate the need for new services.

Benefits to Managed Care Professionals

- An intelligent mix of physicians and nurses results in the most cost-effective care.
- Empowering nurses to make decisions at the patient level reduces bureaucracy.
- Nurse case managers promote a variety of patient choices.

■ Excellent customer service by nurses raises the profitability of managed care.

■ Nurses build positive relationships with your providers.

Using Smart Nursing to Achieve These Benefits

Smart Nursing strategies can potentially improve the work environment in all types of health care organizations. They provide a solid foundation to develop a culture based on positive and respectful relationships.

Accountability is a form of respect. When you hold nurses accountable for results and delegate enough decision-making authority to them, they can do their best work.

Some facilities are capitalizing on using nursing knowledge and the consistency of nursing's presence by using nurses as advisors to physicians. An article in *Modern Healthcare* (Morrissey, 2002) describes how some medical facilities are using nurse specialists to coach doctors regarding effective medical protocol:

> It's not unusual for a nurse to approach a physician at Hackensack [NJ] University Medical Center and talk about the right clinical steps to take on behalf of a patient. Surprisingly, it's not unusual for the doctor to take direction from the nurse. But it's for an unusually good reason. The impact of this collegial exchange, and the program that encourages it, is so evident at the 635-bed hospital that the practice of using clinically specialized nurses to monitor and prompt doctors is becoming routine in cardiac and pulmonary care, where the approach was first tried during the past few years [. . .] The benefits for hospital operations include dramatically higher compliance with proven standards of clinical treatment, along with business bonuses that include lower cost per case and the opportunity to earn millions in extra revenue by improving outcomes and freeing up beds faster. (Morrissey, 2002)

So why do some doctors continue to treat nurses with disrespect? According to another article in *Modern Healthcare* (Tieman, 2002), more than 30% of nurses knew a nurse who had quit because of poor treatment by a physician. This information is based on a study by the Voluntary Hospital of America (VHA).

According to Ronstein (cited in Tieman, 2002), 92% of respondents said they had witnessed disruptive physician behavior, such as inappropriate conflict involving verbal or even physical abuse of nurses. All of the respondents identified a direct link between such behavior and nurse recruitment and retention challenges. Yelling and "condescending behavior" constituted the vast majority of the abuse that doctors inflict on their nurse colleagues (Tieman, 2002).

Physicians have traditionally used interactions with nurses as a way to vent their stress. This is no more right than parents who try to relieve stress by abusing their children. Anyone victimizing another person is wrong. Physicians need to find more mature stress-relief measures.

This treatment of nurses decreases physician success. Suppose a patient overhears her doctor speaking rudely to an office nurse. Don't you think that the patient lowers her opinion of that doctor as a result? Disrespectful behavior interferes with patient-physician relationships and may even lead to litigation.

Physician liability costs have escalated. Respectful treatment of others may reduce this liability. Nurses reduce physician liability because they frequently notify physicians about complications before their patients experience permanent disability or die. You could hire an extra nurse and pay his or her salary for 100 years before you reach $5 million—a common award in medical liability suits (calculated by using $50,000 as the nurse's salary).

Another reason for nurses and physicians to treat each other with respect is because they share a common problem. Both have lost control of their practices, resulting in a new professional dilemma: not enough time to provide adequate patient care. Several physicians have asked me to include some ideas for them in this book because many physicians have become just as disenchanted with the health care system as nurses have. Perhaps physician dissatisfaction is one cause for the negative treatment of nurses.

How Physicians Can Raise Their Own Satisfaction Level

1. Work as partners with other health care staff.
2. Combine your strength to push for positive change.
3. Reduce your liability by listening to other health care professionals.
4. Empower and support nurses. This enables you to reduce some of your own responsibilities.
5. Support advanced practice nurses (legislation increasing their autonomy). Advance practice nurses add to your own success.
6. Working cooperatively with nurses is energy enhancing; conflict is energy draining.
7. Achieve superior patient-care outcomes using synergy, achieving better work in a group than working individually.

How Physicians Can Improve Nurse Satisfaction

1. Genuinely respect nurses as important professionals. More than 75% of communication is nonverbal. Unless you feel genuine respect, your body language will display your true feelings.
2. Educate yourself about nursing. Physicians often aren't aware of what nurses are capable of and what nurses legally can and cannot do. Familiarize yourself with your state's nurse-practice act so that you know what nurses are legally allowed to do. Many physicians take nurses for granted and don't value their work.
3. Appreciate nurses. Nurses are an extra pair of eyes and ears for physicians. Observant nurses warn physicians about impending patient complications in time to prevent death or permanent disability. Show appreciation by using nurse assessments. Give appropriate praise for nurses who do their jobs well.
4. Communicate with courtesy. Nurses need respectful communication to achieve excellent performance. It's time to break the old habits of superiority. It's time to consider nurses as equals.
5. Use nursing data. Patient care suffers when nursing input is ignored. We can no longer continue to make errors caused by reluctance to consider all of the patient data.

Consider the following example of a physician using nursing data to improve patient care: A nurse notices that a psychiatric patient appears anxious. He reviews her medications and notices that she has medication available to relieve her anxiety. However, he also notices that the dosage, although not harmful, would probably cause this patient to sleep much of the day, interfering with her ability to attend therapy groups. He contacts the physician and requests a lower dosage of the medication so that his patient can relieve her anxiety but also attend groups.

As health care workplaces become more respectful, patients will enjoy improved care. My hope is that patients and caregivers will find new ways to work together.

Smart Nursing Strategies for Non-Nurses

Patient Safety

Non-nurses can use Smart Nursing core values to maximize these assets. Respect, flexibility, simplicity, culture, integrity, communication, and caring are all good tools for non-nurses. An added advantage is that these strategies are free of charge.

What some non-nurses have found difficult is eliminating some of health care's sacred cows. We must abandon our rigid hierarchical system, which places physicians and managers high above the frontline employees such as nurses. We must utilize all of the best information, whether the source of that information is a physician, a nurse, or a manager. And we must learn to communicate with each other with courtesy and respect.

Daniel Goleman (2002) shares the following example of how CEO and physician attitudes can actually increase medical errors:

> They don't have enough real contact with people in their organizations. [. . .] These leaders are clueless, or in denial about the reality of their organization. While they may believe that everything is fine, they have in fact created a culture in which no one dares to tell them anything that might provoke them, especially bad news. That kind of silence can come at a very high price.
>
> One physician [. . .] told us: "In the culture of hospitals, a nurse who corrects a doctor—telling him he wrote too many zeroes in an order for patient's meds—can get her head bitten off. If medicine were to adopt the zero tolerance for mistakes that sets the norm for the airline mechanic industry, we'd cut medical errors drastically." (Goleman, 2002)

Nurses complained all through the 1990s that short staffing was unsafe. And they were absolutely right. The large research studies described in the Introduction to this book have determined that even one patient added to a nurse's assignment greatly increases the medical error rate.

Our fast-paced health care environment requires quick responses. Nurses would be able to decrease some of their medical errors if they were allowed to take quick actions to prevent injury. Consider the following perspective about power and how Alan Weiss views the relationship between powerlessness and bureaucracy:

> There is a grand myth extant in organizational life that "power corrupts," a vestige of an overzealous reading of Edmund Burke 200 years ago. Actually, the opposite position is true in business: powerlessness corrupts.
>
> When employees are truly powerless—that is, they cannot make decisions which influence the outcome of their work—they will create artificial power.

Psychologically, most people can't remain healthy if they are engaged in a job, which they routinely cannot influence. This is a sometimes desperate and always encumbering attempt to control their environment and bring some influence to their work lives.

What we encounter as customers are ridiculous policies, rude comments, harsh treatment and deliberate sabotage. That's because employees who feel powerless create artificial power, which we generally refer to as "bureaucracy." (Weiss, 2000)

Non-nurses achieve more success when they examine the following three aspects of their organizations: structure, process, outcomes.

Structure

Analyze the formal and informal power structures in your organization. Ask yourself, "Who actually has the power?" Think about whether a simplified structure would improve outcomes. Would you benefit by building in more flexibility so that you can respond to rapid industry changes? Does your structure help or hinder your customers' well-being? What about your corporate values? Are they a practical guide or merely abstractions?

Process

Do you suffer from bureaucratic gridlock? Would sensible downsizing allow you to function better? Consider whether simplifying procedures would streamline your processes without decreasing quality. How could employee autonomy help? Are you satisfied with your employee performance? What kinds of controls do you have in place? What are your strategies to stimulate innovation by frontline employees? Do your employees exhibit critical-thinking skills?

Outcomes

What is your safety record? What scores have you achieved in patient satisfaction surveys? Are you profitable? Is your profitability consistent? If not, why not? Do you produce a quality product or service? Are your employees satisfied? What is your employee turnover rate? Would your employees recommend your organization to others? Overall, would you describe your outcomes as progress or regress?

Look inward. Look at your structures, processes, and outcomes. Then use the Smart Nursing core values and guiding principles to make improvements.

Consumer Issues

Patient satisfaction is related to profitability, because a good reputation is what attracts patients.

Many times, people meeting nurses give feedback about their medical issues. For example, consider the following experience that a fellow professional shared with me during a conference: He was fighting depression and went to his primary physician, who responded by prescribing an antidepressant. "It's quicker to write a prescription than to talk," the physician explained. "I don't have enough time for an adequate dialogue." This physician was most likely caught up in the vicious cycle of caring for too many patients without enough time to provide quality care.

Patients need consistency. Warm bonds with caregivers are healing in and of themselves. Consistency and relationships enable staff members to do a better job. Caregivers lose effectiveness without a good understanding about a patient's personality, family, and personal values.

Medically complex procedures and lifesaving technologies do not replace the basic human need for love, caring, and compassion. Infants consistently become physically ill and even die if they receive only physical care, without hearing the voice or feeling the touch of a parent or other caring person. Human beings continue to have these needs throughout their lives.

Regardless of one's beliefs, people need spiritual as well as physical care. Recent data have suggested that our brains are wired for some form of spirituality. Various types of exercise, yoga, and even martial arts have been used for years to promote health. The parent of a child who won a contest to see who could stack the most Oreo cookies attributed his child's heightened sense of concentration to his Tai Chi training. Studies about friendship describe its important health benefits for people of all ages. Some health care organizations have started promoting prayer. Meditation has been used for years to promote better physical and mental health.

Some organizations try to pass nonreimbursed health care costs on to the uninsured. These patients—the working poor, the unemployed, young adults, or the self-employed—are the least able to bear this burden.

The ease of international travel has enabled global epidemics and medication-resistant organisms to become more dangerous. Pharmaceutical company policies and high prices make it difficult for the average person to discriminate between price gouging and legitimate costs of research. World poverty, political conflict, and the need to share health resources beyond national borders complicate these issues even more.

As Baby Boomers age, fewer nurses will be present to care for greater needs. This crunch will only get worse. Some reports indicate that we have enough nurses, but nurses have been driven out of health care by negative workplace environments.

Consumers have access to the Internet, which provides an abundance of medical information, yet the average consumer is unable to understand the data fully. They frequently aren't able to prioritize this information accurately or to use it to make intelligent decisions. On the positive side, the Web is an important health-promotion tool. Consumers have used the Internet to assist their physicians with their care. Some families of patients with rare diseases have spent many hours researching information on the Web and have found lifesaving treatment protocols for their loved ones. Many physicians use Internet information for patient education. They refer specific sites as good sources for information about disease and medication. The Web is a good source of health care research because there is an abundance of information available, but one of the biggest problems to avoid is information overload.

Managed Care: Having It All—Safety, Quality, and Cost Control

Consumers need the benefits that managed care (MC) organizations offer. More collaboration between medical professionals, consumers, and related health care industries would strengthen the whole health care system.

Managed care would be the most promising way to resolve our health care challenges—if it achieved its full potential. At present, MC has the opportunity to capitalize on economies of scale—with money, knowledge, and technology. Managed care organizations (MCOs) could provide the highest quality of care for the lowest possible cost. But they fail to do so.

We have changed from a fee-for-service system to a capitated system, whereby organizations assume risks for the total care needs for a specific number of people for a fixed amount of money. As with any service business, MCOs were expected to provide a service in return for payments by employers, individuals, and governmental agencies.

One of the problems that occurred is that some MCOs tried to minimize the service that they provided and maximize the payments that they received. It's no different than a restaurant watering down its soup and losing its loyal customers, and it didn't take long for MCOs to lose consumer trust.

As a result, MC has become a nightmare for many people. A 2003 Gallup poll asked people what they thought were the most honest and respected professions. "Car salesman scored lowest in this year's poll, followed by HMO managers" (AHA, 2003). Because nurses were rated the highest, at 83%, and MC managers were rated next to last, perhaps MC managers should ask nurses how to interact with customers and raise their score.

Effective MC

Effective MC could provide invaluable services to consumers:

- Listening to patients
- Promoting preventative care
- Reducing expensive acute care
- Providing quality outcomes
- Individualizing care
- Focusing on high-touch as well as high-tech care
- Providing superior customer service
- Maintaining cost controls

Consider how MC broadens access to health care services:

1. Access to lifesaving care is available for patients who would otherwise find cutting-edge health care out of their reach. For example, a young couple, just starting out with a new home and new jobs, give birth to a baby who needs care that totals $100,000. They would never have been able to provide this care without health insurance (MC).
2. Access is available to skilled professionals who have the knowledge to guide patients through the illness process. For instance,

an MC company assigns a case manager and health coach to a patient suffering from heart failure. Through teaching and medication management, this patient is able to reduce her emergency room visits by 50% over a 12-month period. She enjoys a higher level of health for the year, and her MC company was able to reduce its costs.

3. Access is available to preventative care that is not only cost-effective for treating disease but also provides patients with a higher quality of life. Smokers have access to smoking cessation programs to improve their quality of life and reduce long-term medical costs.

4. Access to research enables patients to benefit from innovative treatments. A young child is able to receive a new treatment for cancer that saves his life. Research used by MC has made this possible.

5. Access is available to physicians who collaborate with skilled specialists, nurse practitioners, case managers, nurses, and other professionals. The MCOs can provide multidisciplinary care management. For example, a patient who was injured at work receives medical case-management services and advice from an orthopedic specialist. She recovers 25% faster and returns to work two weeks earlier.

When MC Fails

1. An MCO denies preventive care and ends up paying much more for high acute-care costs. An MCO denies weight-reduction treatment for an obese patient who is later hospitalized several times for cardiac conditions that could have been prevented by the weight loss.

2. An MCO takes so long to approve care that the patient's medical condition becomes worse. The resulting cost is twice what it would have been with timely approval. For example, a patient is denied hospital admission for a psychiatric illness. The illness escalates and the MCO ends up paying more: high costs for an ER visit in addition to major hospitalization costs.

3. The MCO strays from its mission of providing quality service to patients and denies as many services as possible. Many states have passed laws that require maternity patients to have 48 hours

of hospitalization instead of leaving after only 24 hours. Government intervention should never have been necessary.

4. An MCO denies alternative medicine measures that have been effective for certain patients. Suppose that a patient finds relief from a spinal injury with acupuncture, but her MCO refuses coverage. She loses many workdays because other treatment has not been effective for her. Her acupuncture is less expensive than covered services, but it is still denied.

5. Unrealistic pressure on physicians to speed up their care reduces their ability to provide adequate treatment. Consider a physician who finds that he is unable to provide patients with even a minimum of quality care. He must see too many patients per hour. This caring physician retires early because his strong professional values about quality care remain unmet. Health care consumers have lost another well-qualified physician.

6. Inconsistent communication results in patient inconvenience. A patient needs care but has to spend many hours on the phone to ensure that his bills are paid. This interferes with his work hours and reduces his productivity.

7. The MCO may be serving the bureaucracy instead of serving the patient: with little accountability to serve patients, the MCO staff talk with patients who call but keep transferring them from department to department without resolving any of their issues.

8. The MCOs use a coercive approach to providers and prevent them from receiving fair reimbursement. Patients lose their local providers and have to drive long distances to other physicians and hospitals. If the contract that is offered to providers reimburses at such a low rate that the provider loses money on each patient, the provider may pull out of the contract. Many patients have to drive long distances to another provider.

Many non-nurses never realized the importance of nursing until so many departed from the health care industry. They never understood the real nature of nursing work until it remained undone. Now is a good time to become knowledgeable about nursing and to learn how to integrate nurses into health care effectively.

Promoting Collaboration With Other Professionals and With Patients

TIPS FOR CLINICAL NURSES

- Understand the CEO perspective.
- Build nurse-physician partnerships.
- Listen to what patients are saying.
- Read minutes of senior management's meetings if available.
- Look for ways to support positive MC initiatives.

TIPS FOR MANAGERS

- Support nurse and non-nurse collaboration.
- Communicate organizational vision to staff.
- Promote alignment of different management levels.
- Point out nursing's key role to organizational success.
- Assess employee attitudes.

TIPS FOR EDUCATORS

- Include cost issues in your curriculum.
- Update your own knowledge about non-nurse issues.
- Dialogue with MC professionals.
- Be open-minded.
- Encourage students to look at the big picture.

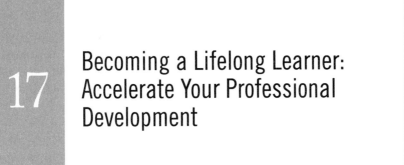

17 Becoming a Lifelong Learner: Accelerate Your Professional Development

Learners will inherit the earth while the learned will be wonderfully equipped to deal with a world that no longer exists. —*Eric Hoffer*

Lifelong learning prepares nurses who are able to thrive in a constantly changing environment. Consider two universal truths: knowledge is power and, when you stop learning, you stop living.

Students are our future. New nurses will have an opportunity to determine the future of nursing by examining our system with fresh eyes. After training, they will be able to introduce new perspectives and needed reform. Will our nursing education programs fulfill this promise? It is an awesome responsibility.

Review the following statement from Dennis O'Leary, MD, past president of the Joint Commission, who took the following position on health care staffing and safety during his testimony before the Senate Committee on Governmental Affairs in June of 2003:

> This country is neglecting to concomitantly improve the professional education system to support the new thinking about prevention of errors and adverse events in this complex delivery system. We need to graduate health care professionals who are proficient in "systems thinking," who are comfortable using decision support tools, and who can actively engage in solving patient safety problems (The Joint Commission, 2003).

Students: Assess your nursing program by asking the following questions:

1.   Does your nursing program encourage independent thinking?
2.   Are you encouraged to use problem-solving strategies from other professions? For example, do you look at the methods that engineers or marketing professionals use and compare them to health care approaches?
3.   What communication and persuasive skills do you learn?
4.   Are change management skills included in your curriculum?
5.   When encouraged to maintain high standards, does your program give you specific ways about how you can accomplish this when you are assigned many more patients after graduation?
6.   Are you encouraged to study politics and group dynamics?
7.   What experiences with other disciplines do you have? Do you know how other industries handle safety, customer satisfaction, and leadership? Have you talked with physical therapists, dieticians, and other health care professionals about the best ways to work together?
8.   Are you encouraged to engage in self-reflection?
9.   Is your critical thinking supported?
10. Are you learning leadership and management skills?

Health care needs nurse-education programs that prepare new graduates who are able to function well in their first jobs. Many health care facilities provide internships to assist new graduates in this transition. Internships have been a successful trend, but they operate better when new graduates come already well prepared.

Students need nursing instructors who are clinical role models and expert nurses themselves. The best nursing programs form cooperative partnerships with a variety of clinical facilities: medical centers, nursing homes, adult day care centers, community health clinics, visiting nurse associations (VNAs), and others. This arrangement provides many mutual advantages. The clinical facilities enrich their practice, and the nurse education programs profit from ready access to outstanding clinical experiences.

Clinical experience is extremely important because it forms the basis for making smart clinical decisions. There are two ways to measure clinical experience. Suppose you meet a nurse with 10 years of experience. You need to decide whether that nurse has one year of experience repeated 10 times or actually has 10 years of experience.

Having 10 years of experience means that you have been willing to step out of your comfort zone whenever you have had an opportunity to learn. You have used Smart Nursing core values and guiding principles to see yourself as an asset to be developed. And you have looked at your work from a long-term perspective.

This will enable you to exhibit excellent clinical judgment by using valuable clinical intuition. These skills are important to maintaining a solid patient safety record because they enable you to make clinical decisions in a timely way.

Magnet Force 14: Professional Development

The health care organization values and supports the personal and professional growth and development of staff. In addition to quality orientation and in-service education, as addressed earlier in Magnet Force 11, Nurses as Teachers, emphasis is placed on career development services. Programs that promote formal education, professional certification, and career development are evident. Competency-based clinical and leadership-management development is promoted, and adequate human and fiscal resources for all professional development programs are provided (ANCC).

How Experts Become Experts

Do experts have greater innate ability, or do people become experts through training and experience? Researchers found that people can usually contemplate only five to nine items at a time. The difference between novices and experts is that novices retrieve five to nine items of information from long-term memory, but an expert quickly retrieves five to nine chunks of information from long-term memory to working memory. There may be 25 or more items in each chunk, so an expert may contemplate 225 items in his or her working memory (9×25), compared to 9 items for a novice. According to the researchers, "the preponderance of psychological evidence indicates that experts are made, not born" (Ross, 2006).

What does this mean for nurses who are on the path to becoming an expert nurse? Suppose you are a charge nurse, and a patient seems to be developing some disturbing symptoms. The reality of patient care is that you don't have the luxury of waiting to obtain all of the data that you might need. For example, you must make a decision before you have all the lab test results. You must decide whether to wait and assess further, report the symptoms to the physician, or operate in an emergency mode. Experienced clinical nurses are usually able to decide on the correct action to take.

If you are a new nurse, this is a good time to consult with an experienced nurse, to add to your personal "database of clinical experience" so that you will eventually become an experienced nurse. Every nurse was a beginner at some point and went through the same process.

The secret of fast learning is to volunteer to learn as much as possible. Volunteer to become IV certified; work to become certified in your specialty; plan to become advanced cardiac life support (ACLS) certified, if that designation is relevant to your work. Ask relevant questions. Volunteer to cross-train, or develop a staff or patient education program. Take the initiative. Step outside your comfort zone. Develop a reputation of one who is consistently seeking professional growth. As you reach professional milestones, give yourself a reward.

Not all employers value experienced nurses. If that is the case, you can set up your own coaching strategy, educate your employer using Smart Nursing core values and guiding principles, or look for another job where your professional growth will be supported. Experienced nurses sometimes resist this coaching role, because it takes extra time, but accepting this role makes experienced nurses valuable to their organization. Experienced nurses also find that teaching novice nurses sharpens their own skills; teaching requires nurses to review the rationale of their practices. Smart organizations reward experienced nurses who are willing to coach others.

Many organizations use a system of clinical ladders to recognize higher levels of nursing excellence. With this approach, nurses with excellent clinical skills do not have to seek out management positions to earn more money and recognition. Most organizations recognize three levels of expertise, and the role of Clinical Nurse III usually includes staff coaching, an expanded patient teaching role, and an expectation of solid critical-thinking skills.

Learn Strategies for Change

Look at your work environment to see how it could be better. Notice who is influential in your organization, and observe how they became effective. Make the following observations:

1. Do people introduce suggestions at staff meetings? Are they successful? What communication approach do they use?

2. Do they talk formally or informally with the nurse manager?
3. Do people put their requests in writing?
4. Do they seek out coworkers with similar perspectives and make suggestions as a group?
5. Have they presented suggestions at open meetings with the CEO? Were they effective?

Once you understand how successful change happens at your workplace, you will know what to do. Use your assessment and planning skills to become an effective change agent.

When you make a job change, start the observation process again; the politics at each facility are different. In each new job, spend at least three months observing how the new system works. Even positive cultures have personalities; they have certain ways to get things done. It is not a matter of good or bad; it's a matter of learning how your organization works. This observation method will enable you to identify quickly the strategies that successful people use in that setting.

The Value of Intellectual Capital

Intellectual capital is one of your organization's most valuable assets, and it keeps on growing if managed well. We live in the information age. Nurses are part of their organization's capital. How you develop your skill sets determines how much value you have to offer. If you use this currency well, your facility will become intellectually wealthy. Intellectual capital includes work experience, specialized training, natural aptitudes, non-nursing experience, and creativity.

Review the skills assessment in the Appendix for a list of attributes that are important to personal and professional effectiveness. Broad skills enable nurses to become qualified clinicians, managers, and leaders. Skills that are especially important to influence others are public speaking, writing for publication, networking, and activity in professional associations. Articulate nurses are more likely to be heard.

The silence of nurses has been one of the main reasons for the nursing crisis. We have expected others to speak for us. No one has. We must find our voice and start speaking for ourselves.

Health care is a rapidly changing industry. Nurses who are avid students are able to retain their competency. You don't even have to enroll in an education program. Educate yourself by doing the following:

- Cultivate a sense of curiosity.
- Ask questions. When you meet other people, people from other industries as well, ask them how they approach their challenges. Then use an open mind to see if you can apply their techniques in health care.
- Go to your local library at least once a month.
- Check out a dozen books on a variety of subjects, and set aside a couple of hours to skim through them.
- Look for good ideas.
- Read a few chapters from your favorite books.

My experience has been that you will find something useful for health care in every single book. You will also be a good role model in lifelong learning for your peers and children.

Our world has changed, and so have the rules of the game. People have enjoyed long-term security in the past by working for the same organization. Now, the number of skills that you are able to exercise determines your job security, so your job security resides with you. Most important, because you have control of how many skills you learn, job security is an internal instead of an external issue.

- Be proactive. Anticipate and embrace change rather than waiting to be forced. Rapid changes of census and acuity make cross-training a fact of life. You have two choices: embrace cross-training and learn to do it well (positive) or complain each time that your assignments change (negative).
- Brainstorm with your peers to identify emerging trends.
- Identify certain skills that have a particularly high return for your effort: Advanced Cardiac Life Support certification, IV certification, adult learning theory, Cardiopulmonary Resuscitation (CPR) instructor certification, and communication, leadership and management skills.
- Empower yourself with effective communication.
- Learn everything you can. When an opportunity to learn a new skill surfaces, volunteer right away. Accepting free training is always a smart decision. Become multiskilled as soon as possible.

- Expand your people skills so that you can function as an effective team leader. Listen to your team members with sensitivity.
- Notice superb team leaders and observe how they interact with their team members.
- Read publications from both health care and non-health care industries. Broaden your perspective by exchanging information between disciples.
- Capitalize on diversity.

Consider the following example of successfully combining diverse viewpoints using education: An educator, who was asked to plan a program on innovation, decided to organize a panel that included four teams. Each team was composed of a natural innovator paired up with an influential long-term staff member. This exercise strengthened both people. The innovator became more influential and the long-term nurse more innovative, and the staff in the audience gained from the variety of participant perspectives.

Information from different industries and disciplines has common foundations. A breadth of knowledge enables you to apply basic ideas in a variety of different ways. Use the following ideas to broaden your perspective:

- Ask "Why?" when you do something new.
- Then ask, "Does it make sense?"
- Think about ways to accomplish your work more simply while still achieving good results.
- Ask yourself if you have considered all of the possibilities. Talk with others to determine whether they see situations differently.
- Cultivate an appreciation of novel thoughts and perspectives.
- Become a role model for personal and professional growth.
- Believe in yourself. Expect resistance from the status quo. Learn not to take negative feedback personally.
- Network (network everywhere).
- Cultivate an appreciation for other people.
- Develop expertise in small talk.
- Find good role models and learn from them.
- Limit your television-watching time and use it for reading instead.
- Keep books in your car and read while you wait for appointments or wait to pick up your children.
- Read for 30 minutes every morning. That adds up to more than three hours of reading every week. And it makes your day more focused.

As experienced patient interviewers, nurses already possess communication skills. They just need to reconfigure those communication skills to make them more versatile.

Health care is a labor-intensive industry, and money spent on human resources constitutes a large portion of a health care organization's budget. Staff development directors have an opportunity to leverage this large investment with strategic education programs.

Health care organizations need large numbers of competent nurses. They need nurses who are flexible, good at working in fast-paced environments, and competent in a wide variety of clinical areas. They need nurses who advocate for patient safety.

Imagine the difference in health care organizations if nurses were more assertive and articulate. What if nurses wrote articles, spoke to community groups, and influenced health care policies. Collectively, we have the knowledge, information, and compassion needed for health care reform.

BEST PRACTICE: INTEGRATING EVIDENCE INTO NURSING'S CULTURE: TRANSFORMATION OF THE NURSING EDUCATION DEPARTMENT

Susan Hoolahan, RN, MSN, CNAA-BC, Vice President of Patient Care Services, CNO, University of Pittsburgh Medical Center, UPMC-St Margaret, Pittsburgh, PA
Jacqueline O'Brien, MSN, RN, CIC, Director of Nursing Education, University of Pittsburgh Medical Center, UPMC-St Margaret, Pittsburgh, PA.

We transformed our traditional nursing education department into a flexible model that integrated evidence into clinical practice. The content of our education programs changed from competency and orientation programs to using APNs (Advanced Practice Nurses) with strong foundations in Evidence-Based Practice (EBP) and research to support bedside clinicians in posing questions, reviewing literature, and seeking better outcomes for their patients. University of Pittsburgh Medical Center-St. Margaret is a 250-bed community teaching hospital, part of a large integrated health care system.

Key decisions that led to our success were:

■ Hiring a director of nursing education to redesign the department.
■ Changing from a convenience model to one based on skill sets and clinical expertise.

- Assigning clinical hours to each APN-nurse educator with clearly defined responsibilities, new hire support, assessment and observation, and integration of EBP into clinical decision making.
- Preparation of the educators to share the message of EBP.

We utilized a behavioral leadership questionnaire to assess work satisfaction (qualitatively) and a team empowerment tool. The results were an improved team and behavioral leadership and anecdotal unit evidence demonstrating a strong relationship between the educators' increased presence and successful new hire management, problem solving, and dissemination of information.

The traditional education room was refurbished to create an atmosphere that is facilitative to learning and gives the impression to all who enter that St. Margaret truly loves and values its nurses. This room is used for orientation, continuing education, and meetings to collaborate with other nurses.

Comments from unit clinicians:

"I love this room. I spend four hours here a week."

"Wow. All who come here will feel supported."

"Congratulations on developing a truly calming and relaxing space for learning."

Resistance encountered: fear of change, the unfounded fear of job loss, fear of role and responsibility change, and fear of conducting research. We managed resistance by utilizing evidence to support all decision making and by believing in positive outcomes.

Conclusion

Nursing education processes, methods, and content should follow the evolution of nursing practice toward EBP by devoting valuable resources from nursing administration as support.

Promoting for Lifelong Learning

TIPS FOR CLINICAL NURSES

- Think strategically.
- Look for opportunities.
- Keep your sense of humor.
- Learn from your mistakes.
- Cross-train.

TIPS FOR MANAGERS

- Support nurses' professional growth.
- Recognize that nurses are high-value human resources.
- Consider nurses as assets.
- Encourage knowledge sharing.
- Support nurses who step out of their comfort zone.

TIPS FOR EDUCATORS

- Involve students in discussions about working with LPNs, LNA/CNAs, and others.
- Build student self-confidence.
- Discuss self-development challenges.
- Promote flexibility.
- Encourage students to take intelligent risks.

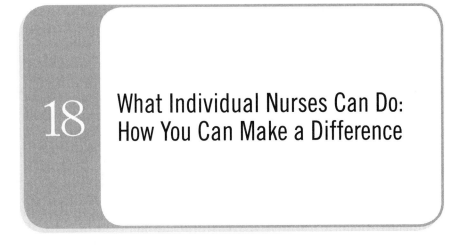

18 What Individual Nurses Can Do: How You Can Make a Difference

The best way to get what you want is to help the other side get what they want. —*Robert Shapiro*

Look at the Big Picture

Help management get what it wants so that nurses can get what they want. Conflict between nurse and management is needless, expensive, and wasteful. Worst of all, it consumes time, talent, and money that is needed for direct-patient care.

Nurses and administrators share responsibility for this problem, but, because this chapter focuses primarily on clinical nurses, it points out how they can impact the nursing crisis by changing something about themselves.

Enlarge your thinking to include your CEO's viewpoint. You already know from communicating with patients that you must frame clinical suggestions around patient issues. Use the same principle when working with management—frame your requests around their important issues: safety, marketing, and financial success.

CEOs are responsible for organizations' survival. Issues that CEOs frequently consider to be important are (a) balancing the budget—many payers reimburse less than the actual cost of care—(b) expanding health care services into new markets; and (c) minimizing medical errors and risk.

Reframe Your Perspectives

Frame your comments from an articulate business point of view. Show how nursing adds value to your organization. Suppose you work at a small community hospital with a wonderfully compassionate and competent nursing staff. An outstanding neurosurgeon from a nearby metropolitan area prefers to admit his patients to your hospital, mainly because of nursing excellence. Consider yourself as an important partner when talking with management. Comment on the value that nurses bring to the organization.

CEOs are beginning to realize that having enough good nurses is necessary for survival. This is new realization, because nurses have been undervalued in the past.

Point out that excellent patient care is an important factor that attracts patients to your facility. Patients tend to listen to their friends and neighbors when choosing health care facilities. Capitalize on that trend. Calculate your spin-off value as a premier marketer.

- Patients who are highly satisfied by their nursing care bring millions of dollars of revenue later on by recommending your facility to their friends and neighbors. And they are likely to return if they have further medical needs.
- Suppose a patient asks for a more homelike atmosphere in the hospital. This information is valuable input for management.
- Communicate a negative situation if it exists. Say, "The current short staffing is driving our patients away. Something needs to be done. We can't afford to keep losing patients. And, if the staffing remains low, we will be losing many nurses as well."

Look for Ways to Add Value to Your Organization

It is important to communicate this kind of information to your CEO and other managers. Focus on building bridges to a better future instead of just repeating the past.

- Seek out councils, committees, or boards created to obtain nursing ideas.

- Initiate conversations with your vice president of nursing to share mutual perspectives.
- Talk with committee members. Examine written records, and analyze their goals and actions.
- Inquire about joining an interdisciplinary group, such as a customer satisfaction group that is composed of many disciplines. Raise patient satisfaction by building relationships with a variety of professionals.
- Improve your communication skills so that you can effectively add substance to discussions. Learn negotiation skills so that you can be a player instead of a spectator.
- Focus on improving your critical-thinking skills so that your suggestions become advances into the future instead of retreats into the past.
- Make a suggestion about new ways to help your organization's success.

Initiate Partnerships With Management

Partnerships only work when management views nurses as valued professionals. Make the first move and build mutual respect.

I enrolled in my first business course, Accounting I, in 1983. My peers were surprised and wondered why a nurse working at a non-profit health care facility would want to take an accounting course. They implied that a clinical nurse should focus only on clinical nursing issues. They thought that nurses should leave the business side of health care to management. My perspective was different. I took accounting because my focus was on clinical issues. And my focus is still on clinical care. Improving patient care is one of my main reasons for writing this book.

Nurses cannot provide patients with adequate care unless they have enough resources—enough employees, supplies, and support staff. Part of our job is to communicate patient needs to management effectively. We must speak the language of business, articulate clinical needs, and understand our scarce resource environment.

Be Business Savvy

Nurses must be business savvy to obtain the necessary financial resources that drive quality care. Learning the language of business is a good first step. When staffing is inadequate, point out—in business terms—that your facility can no longer afford the financial loss caused by short staffing. Consider the following suggestions:

- Short staffing causes nurses to find other jobs or leave the health care industry for good. Every time a nurse resigns, management loses more than $50,000.
- Short staffing increases the number of medical errors and raises your risk.
- Nurses are your greatest asset. Value them and treat them with respect.

Non-health care organizations have succeeded by supporting the autonomy of frontline employees. Frontline employees are entrusted with the responsibility of satisfying the customers because they have the most customer contact. They become ambassadors for their companies. Companies who promote staff autonomy have been successful over time.

Be Accountable

Many nurses understandably are reluctant to accept greater account-ability. They have been censured in the past for challenging the status quo, and they are reluctant to try again. But we must try again. Nurse autonomy is absolutely necessary if we hope to succeed in controlling health care costs and reducing medical errors. If management refuses to promote nurse autonomy, clinical nurses must educate manage-ment and be willing to demonstrate the benefits to their organiza-tion. Combine your clinical knowledge with solid persuasive skills to make sure that your recommendations to improve patient care are implemented.

Look to the future instead of repeating past practices. The nurs-ing crisis may end up being just the right catalyst to transform health care problems into opportunities and actually improve health. Welcome difficult challenges. Nurses often engage in subtle avoidance behavior. They get sidetracked when confronted with problems. Instead of solving the main problem, they focus on the details first. Focusing on details is important, but first review the basic principles. Ask yourself, "Is this idea logical? Is it ethical? Will it improve patient care? Is it financially sound? Will the staff support it?"

Be Willing to Change

Most progressive people step out of their comfort zones to achieve results. Change feels uncomfortable at first, but that discomfort is soon neutralized by the satisfaction of creating better practice. Use your knowledge and ability to create realistic solutions to health care challenges. Seek out control over your work. Learning new skills—communication, negotiation, and persuasion—will improve patient safety, increase nurse satisfaction, and raise productivity.

Nurses have lost power partly because we have neglected to become excellent communicators and negotiators. We have assumed that others would speak for us. No one has. Nurses are the ones who need to be articulate—learn to speak in public, write for publication, and negotiate effectively.

Join Toastmasters to learn public speaking. You will meet people who had been afraid to speak but have learned how to be well spoken. Join a writers group to learn how to write for publication. Read some books on negotiation. The same is true about writing for publication. A writing course or joining a writers group can enable you to have a second mode to express your views. What are your reasons for waiting? Do you think the process will be too expensive? Most of these organizations are free. Some charge a nominal fee. You just need to act.

Some nurses say that they don't have time. This is understandable, considering the large amount of overtime and other responsibilities. But nurses must take some initiative to stop the cycle of powerlessness and mandatory overtime. Learning new skills to become professionally articulate is the best way to address this vicious cycle.

Cross-Train

Nurses have a huge effect on their organization's financial status because of the size of nursing budgets. Management has constraints from insurers, the government, and others. Nurses need to be flexible and willing to cross-train to help management achieve the best staff utilization. Remember, nurses become more successful when they help their whole organization succeed.

Work in different specialties to broaden your perspective. Network with other nurses and with people in other industries. Read widely. Avoid stagnating and getting in a rut. Be a lifelong learner. Cross-training makes you a better nurse. Medical-surgical nurses who know psychiatry interact better with noncompliant patients or patients with personality disorders. Nurses who understand home care plan better discharges. Ambulatory care nurses with MC experience are better patient advocates. Other cross-training benefits are the following:

- Greater self-confidence
- Higher value to employers
- Better job prospects if you decide to change jobs

Know your limitations about being a safe clinician in new specialties. Be assertive in expressing your concerns if the proposed situation is potentially unsafe for patients or yourself.

Respect Others

Respect the LNA/CNAs. I present education programs to LNA/CNAs as well as to nurses, and I sometimes hear that many nurses do not treat LNA/CNAs well. Are we treating other caregivers the same way that we have been treated? Be good role models. This means that we should use the following guidelines:

- We should treat LNA/CNAs with respect.
- Listen to their perspective. They spend much time with patients and have valuable information.
- Offer to assist LNA/CNAs when they need help. A good way to encourage nurse-LNA/CNA collaboration is to use nurse-LNA/CNA partnerships. Assign a group of patients to nurse-LNA/CNA partnerships. Expect joint accountability. It's time for nurses to value the contribution of all health care workers.
- Take time to teach LNA/CNAs, tactfully and with sensitivity, how to improve their work.
- Use your sense of humor.

Use Tools Sensibly

We have many good tools, but sometimes we sabotage their effectiveness. When carried to the extreme, good tools become liabilities instead of assets. It's similar to the ideas of some patients who sometimes think that if a little bit of medicine is good, a lot must be better. We know that this is not necessarily true. It is the same for nurses. Taking our tools to the extreme turns a positive tool into an obstacle.

Nursing care plans are a perfect example of frequent misuse of a good tool. When care plans were introduced in the 1980s, nurses on each shift either had to ask patients to describe their needs or discover them through an inconsistent reporting system. Many people wanted care plans to have a customized outline. Others wanted them to be more complete and initiated the era of standard care plans. We wrote care plans for every conceivable illness, laminated them, and inserted them into the Kardex. Because the plans were cumbersome and not individualized, nurses did not use them. We wasted a lot of time and money.

Some facilities use a hybrid version of a care plan. It is a simplified guide that includes common nursing interventions for nurses to check off. Blank spaces are available to add interventions that were not included.

Multidisciplinary treatment planning is another good tool that is often misused. In the 1980s, the average psychiatric patient's length of stay was two to three weeks. Now it is often two to three days. However, the treatment-team planning process hasn't changed much. We should be able to write excellent plans in less time. In one case, a nurse was the only one available to care for patients because the rest of the staff were at the treatment-team meeting. Planning is important. But shouldn't our priority be actually giving the care? Effective nursing care plans and multidisciplinary treatment plans represent a significant opportunity to reduce expenses without decreasing quality.

Broaden Your Knowledge

Ideas are the new business capital. We should exchange good ideas among nursing, business, and education on a regular basis. Consider how the following scenarios illustrate the portability of skill sets between health care and other occupations.

A health care sales nurse decided to use SOAP (Subjective, Objective, Assessment, and Plan) notes to write sales reports. These SOAP notes are a clinical charting technique used by nurses and physicians. They are also versatile for many other kinds of reports. The sales manager considered SOAP note sales reports to be the best reports that he had ever received. Compare the medical and sales examples using SOAP notes in Table 18.1.

Table 18.1

	SOAP NOTES	
	Medical example	**Sales example**
S	Patient says, "My stress at work has increased."	Customer says, "We aren't getting our shipments on time."
O	Patient's blood pressure is 150 over 90.	Customer order sheets are correct and faxed on time.
A	There is difficulty coping with company downsizing.	Orders received on Mondays are delayed.
P	Try scheduled rest breaks and exercise for relaxation.	Try rescheduling order-takers on Mondays to avoid shipment delays.

HISTORY OF SOAP NOTES

According to Cameron (2002),

> SOAP notes are part of the problem-oriented medical records (POMR) approach most commonly used by physicians and other health care professionals. Developed by Weed (1964), SOAP notes are intended to improve the quality and continuity of client services by enhancing communication among health care professionals (Ketten-Bach, 1995) and by assisting them in better recalling the details of each client's case (Ryback, 1974; Weed, 1971).

> Critical paths are an example of how information can be transferred from another industry to health care. Critical paths are often considered by health care professionals as a new idea of the 1990s. However, critical paths were adapted for use in health care only after they had been used in other industries for many years. Critical paths were used in engineering for more than 20 years before they were used in health care.

Why don't we transfer information between disciplines more often? Why don't nurses network with people from other industries? If nurses would ask other professionals how they solve their problems, nurses could adapt some of those ideas to health care.

Are you willing to analyze your attitude and behavior? Will you make any necessary changes? Making changes may be easier than you think. And the rewards are great, because it is a well-known fact that people who continue to grow and evolve through their whole lives experience more happiness.

TRACING THE HISTORY OF CRITICAL PATHS

According to Bryant:

> Peg A. Hofman, RN, TQM Coordinator at Mount Clemons General Hospital, traced the beginning of the critical path method [CPM] to the mid-1950s [. . .] At that time annual maintenance projects in the oil and chemical refinery industry were plotted on layouts from start to finish in a timeline that gave a "big picture" visualization.
>
> In industry, it has proven to be a valuable tool for charting projects that require the coordination of hundreds of separate contractors; it is commonly used in engineering, construction, and computer work. The earliest use of CPM reported in health care literature was in the mid-1980s by Zander, who adopted the CPM concept to review the delivery of patient care at the New England Medical Center, in Boston. The technique has been adapted to coordinate projects in both product and service organizations. (Bryant, 1995)

In 1991, Grudich reported a major improvement in operating room efficiency by applying CPM at St. Cloud Hospital in Minnesota. In 1992, the term *critical path* first appeared as a major heading in the index for *Nursing and Allied Literature*.

My question is this: "Why did it take more than 30 years for health care to adopt critical paths?" I think the answer is that health care organizations failed to understand how much they could learn from others.

If health care leaders and clinical workers had networked with those in engineering and the military and with others using critical paths, health care agencies could have enjoyed the benefits of this very useful technique much sooner.

Promoting Individual Nursing Action

TIPS FOR CLINICAL NURSES

- Look at the big picture.
- Be willing to step out of your comfort zone.
- Work toward positive change with your peers.
- Evaluate the effectiveness of your interventions.
- Support your own personal growth.

TIPS FOR MANAGERS

- Encourage clinical nurses to get involved in the change process.
- Value nurse contributions.
- Highlight change efforts by staff nurses on their evaluations.
- Facilitate group efforts for improvements.
- Maximize staff efforts to improve productivity.

TIPS FOR EDUCATORS

- Chart a postgraduate self-development plan.
- Include change management in your curriculum.
- Be forward thinking.
- Support community-building skills.
- Coordinate future needs in your program.

SKILL ASSESSMENT

Mark the skills that you already have with an X. Then circle three skills that you would like to develop. Add other relevant skills and/or qualities in the blank spaces to customize the list.

Learnable/Transferable Skills	Styles to Develop
Public speaking/Networking	Energetic
CPR instructor	Attention to detail
Venipuncture skills	Gets along well with people
Clinical skills (cross-training) Certifications	Determined
Leadership skills	Works well under pressure
Management skills	Sensitive
Conducts research	Intuitive
Storytelling	Persistent
Education theory	Dynamic
Writing	Dependable
Knowledge of legal system	Flexible
Computer competence	Creative/innovative
Efficient reading with comprehension	Problem-solving
Acting	_____
Musical talent	_____
Mediation/diplomacy	_____
Graduate degree	_____
Financial expertise	_____
Strategic planning	_____
_____	_____
_____	_____

References

Aiken, L. H., Clarke, S. P., Silber, J. H., & Sloane, D. (2003, October). Hospital nurse staffing, education, and patient mortality. *LDI Issue Brief, 9*(2), 2–3.

Beurhaus, P., Donelin, D., Ulrich, B., Norman, L., & Dittus, R. (2005). Is the shortage of registered nurses getting better or worse? Findings from two recent national surveys of RNs. *Nursing Economics, 23*(2)(March–April), 58–60.

Brown, M. (1990). *Working ethics: Strategies for decision making and organizations' responsibility.* San Francisco: Jossey-Bass.

Bryant, M. R. (1995). Critical pathways: What they are and what they are not. *Tar Heel Nurse, 57*(5), 18.

Burns, D. (1980). *Feeling good.* New York: Avon Books.

Bylone, M. (2006, January 2). When it comes to preventable medical errors, nurses must take a look at themselves. *ADVANCE for Nurses,* 10.

Cameron, S. (2002). Learning to write case notes using SOAP format. *Journal of Counseling & Development, 80*(3), 2.

Czikszentmihalyi, M. (2004). *Good business.* New York: Penguin.

Dawson, R. (1993). *The confident decision maker.* New York: William Morrow.

Eisler, L. (2007). *The real wealth of nations.* San Francisco: Berrett-Koehler.

Gibson, R., & Prasad Singh, J. (2003). *Wall of silence.* Washington, DC: Lifeline Press.

Goleman, D. (2002). *Primal leadership.* Boston: Harvard Business School Press.

Hawkins, D. (2002). *Power vs. force.* Carlsbad, CA: Hay House.

Hojat, M., & Herman, M. W. (1985). Developing an instrument to measure attitudes toward nurses: Preliminary psychometric findings. *Psychological Reports, 56,* 571–579.

Hughes, R. G., (Ed.). (2008, March). *Patient safety and quality: An evidence-based handbook for nurses.* AHRQ Publication No. 08-0043, prepared with support from the Robert Wood Johnson Foundation. Rockville, MD: Agency for Healthcare Research and Quality.

Jennings, J. (2002). *Less is more.* New York: Penguin Group.

Jessee, W. (2003). It's time for a change. *Modern Healthcare, 33*(41), 26.

Johannes, L. (2002, May 30). Serious health risks posed by lack of nurses. *The Wall Street Journal,* pp. D1, D3.

Jones, C. (2004). The costs of nurse turnover, Part 1: An economic perspective. *The Journal of Nursing Administration, 12*(34), 562–570.

Koch, R. (1998). *The 80/20 principle: The secret of achieving more with less.* New York: Doubleday.

Lancaster, L. (2002). *When generations collide.* New York: Harper Business.

Landau, S., Landau, B., & Landau, D. (2001). *From conflict to creativity: How resolving workplace disagreements can inspire innovation and productivity*. San Francisco: Jossey-Bass.

Loehr, J., & Schwartz, T. (2003). *The power of full engagement*. New York: Free Press.

Maslow, A. (1954). *Motivation and personality*. New York: Harper.

Mitchell, W. (1997). *It's not what happens to you: It's what you do about it*. Denver, CO: Phoenix Press.

Morath, J., & Leary, M. (2004). Creating safe spaces in organizations to talk about safety. *Nursing Economics, 6*(22), 344–354.

Morrissey, J. (2002). Following nurses' orders. *Modern Healthcare, 32*(34), 36.

Needleman, J., Buerhaus, P., Mattke, S., Stewart, M., & Zelevinsky, K. (2002). Nurse staffing levels and the quality of care in hospitals. *New England Journal of Medicine, 346*, 1715–1720.

New York Times. (2002). Editorial: "Dying for lack of nurses." *10*(25).

Nurses Top Gallup's Ethical Standards List. (2003, December 15). *AHA News*, p. 16.

Nursing Executive Center. (2000). *Reversing the flight of talent: Nursing retention in an era of gathering shortage*. Washington, DC: The Advisory Board Company.

Palmer, H., Clanton, M., Ezhuthachan, S., Newman, C., Maisels, J., & Plsek, P. (2003). Applying the "10 Simple Rules" of the Institute of Medicine to hyperbilirubinemia in newborns. *Pediatrics, 112*(6), 1388–1393.

Peck, M. S. (1978). *The road less traveled: A new psychology of love, traditional values, and spiritual growth*. New York: Simon & Schuster.

Pine, R., & Tart, K. (2007). Return on investment: Benefits and challenges of a baccalaureate nurse residency program. *Nursing Economics, 25*(1), 13–18.

Reinhold, B. B. (1996). *Toxic work*. New York: Penguin.

Roane, S. (1997). *What do I say next?* New York: Warner Books.

Ross, P. (2006, August). The expert mind. *Scientific American*, 64–71.

Scott, J. G., Sochalski, J., & Aiken, L. (1999). Review of Magnet hospital research: Findings and implications for professional nursing practice. *Journal of Nursing Administration, 29*(1), 9–19.

Senge, P. (1990). *The fifth discipline: The art and practice of the learning organization*. New York: Doubleday.

Smetzer, J., & Navarra, M. (2007). Measuring change: A key component of building a culture of safety. *Nursing Economics, 25*(1), 49–51.

Spence, G. (1995). *How to argue and win every time*. New York: St. Martin's Press.

Stanley, T. (2000). *The millionaire mind*. Kansas City: Andrews McMeel Publishing.

Tieman, J. (2002). Study: Docs contribute to the nursing shortage. *Modern Healthcare, 32*(24), 26.

Trossman, S. (2006). Preventing errors: IOM report offers strategies throughout the medication process. *The American Nurse, 38*(5), 1, 14.

Tucker, A. L. (2004). The impact of operational failures on hospital nurses and their patients. *Journal of Operations Management 22*, 151–169.

Tucker, A. L., Edmonson, A. C., & Spear, S. (2002). When problem solving prevents organizational learning. *Journal of Organizational Change Management, 15*(2), 135.

Upenieks, V. (2003). What constitutes effective leadership? *Journal of Nursing Administration, 33*, 456–467.

Vogelsmeier, A. (2007). A just culture: The role of nursing leadership. *Journal of Nursing Care Quality, 22*(3), 210–212.

Watson, J. (2005). *Caring science as sacred science.* Philadelphia: F. Davis Company.

Welch, J. (2001). *Jack: Straight from the gut.* New York: Warner Books.

West, J. (2007). Ethical issues and new nurses: Preventing ethical distress in the work environment. *The Kansas Nurse, 82*(4), 5.

Whyte, D. (2001). *Crossing the unknown sea.* New York: Penguin Putnam.

Wilson, E. O. (1998). *Consilience: The unity of knowledge.* New York: Alfred A. Knopf.

Zimbardo, P. (2007). *The Lucifer effect: Understanding how good people turn evil.* New York: Random House.

Zukav, G. (1989). *The seat of the soul.* New York: Fireside Books.

WEB SITES

American Nurse Credentialing Center (ANCC). Forces of magnetism. Retrieved July 2008, from http://www.nursecredentialing.org

American Nurses Association. (2004). ANA staffing guidelines. Retrieved June 2008, from www.needlestick.org/readroom/stffprnc.htm#Recomm

Barsade, S., Ramarajan, L. (2006). What makes the job tough? The influence of organizational respect on burnout in human services. (The Wharton School.) Retrieved July 2008, from http://knowledge.wharton.upenn.edu

Fauntleroy, G. (2007). Hiring one extra RN might help hospitals save lives. (Health Behavior News Service.) Retrieved November 2007, from www.hbns.org

Gallup. (2006). Honesty and ethics. Retrieved July 2008, from www.gallup.com

Institute of Medicine. Keeping patients safe: Transforming the work environment of nurses. Retrieved November 2004, from www.iom.edu

Joint Commission. (June 2003). Patient safety: Instilling hospitals with a culture of continuous improvement. Retrieved December 2004, from www.jointcommission.org

Joint Commission. (July 2008). Joint Commission alert: Stop bad behavior among health care professionals. Retrieved July 2008, from www.jointcommission.org

Kaiser Family Foundation. (2004). Five years after IOM report on medical errors, nearly half of all consumers worry about the safety of their health care. Retrieved October 15, 2008 from www.kff.org

National Patient Safety Foundation. Retrieved July 2008, from www.npsf.org

National Quality Forum. *Safe Practices for Better Health Care.* Retrieved October 2008 from www.qualityforum.org

Needleman, J., Buerhaus, P., Steward, M, et. al. (2006, January 12). Nurse staffing in hospitals: Is there a business case for quality? (the Commonwealth Fund.) Retrieved July 2008, from www.commonwealthfund.org

O'Sullivan, A. Senate Governmental Affairs Committee testimony. (American Nurses Association). Retrieved November 2001, from www.nursingworld.org

Weiss, A. (2000). *Leadership for the new millennium.* Retrieved January 2002, from www.summitconsulting.com

Index